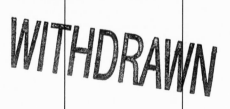

Holistic Oral Care

A Guide for Health Professionals

2nd edition

Janet Griffiths
Associate Specialist
Department of Adult Dental Health
University Dental Hospital
Cardiff
UK

Steve Boyle BDS MSc
Clinical Director of Community Dental Services
Gwent Healthcare NHS Trust
Gwent
UK

2005
Published by Stephen Hancocks Limited
27 Bellamy's Court, Abbotshade Road
London, SE16 5RF
www.shancocksltd.com

ISBN 09546145 2 6

Printed and bound by Dennis Barber Limited. Lowestoft, Suffolk

Preface

Since the publication of the very successful first edition of this book, the context of Special Care Dentistry has changed quite significantly.
We now face the future with the certainty that Special Care Dentistry is here to stay. Whilst the dental profession may take some time more to recognise formal training and accreditation for the dental team, those people responsible for the day to day care of people with disabilities cannot wait. This book aims to address those needs.

This new edition of *Holistic Oral Care* builds on the first edition, by addressing the concerns and needs of a multitude of people, from very different walks of life, who have to carry out the daily business of ensuring that oral health contributes to general well-being as well as enhancing the quality of life for people with impairments.

The contents now reflect a changed world compared with the time when this book was first written. Organising oral and dental care for someone with an impairment has become more complex – issues of access to dental care, judgements on capacity to consent, the minefield surrounding the debate on physical interventions, even before consideration can be given to the increasing choices in clinical dentistry, make the life of the well-intentioned carer so much more difficult.

This book aims to address all these issues in an easy accessible, logical format with guidance from the authors as to how to access the information required. This is a winning formula as testified by the number of reading lists for certificate, diploma and degree courses on which the book appeared. The Preface to the first edition stated that this book was primarily for nurses, other health care professionals and carers; I know that it was read by all these and more. The opportunity that this gives us to really provide holistic team care for vulnerable groups in our society is not to be underestimated.

June Nunn
Dublin, May 2005

Acknowledgements

The first edition of *Holistic Oral Care* would not have been possible without the support of many of our friends and colleagues, and we are eternally grateful for their advice and constructive criticism.

For this second edition, we want to record our appreciation for the support, knowledge and experience of all members of the dental team working in Special Care Dentistry in Wales, to members of the British Society for Disability and Oral Health (BSDH), the International Association of Disability and Oral Health (IADH) and the British Society of Gerodontology (BSG).

Again, our sincere thanks to Frank, Michael, Jo and Edwina in the Dental Illustration Unit at the School of Dentistry at Cardiff University for the their skill and patience. We would also like to thank Debbie and Ruth for all their unstinting help in providing secretarial support throughout the preparation of this edition. And we are most grateful to Professor June Nunn, Editor of the *Journal of Disability and Oral Health* for writing the forward and her encouragement, and the patience of Stephen Hancocks in publishing this edition.

Finally thanks to our respective partners, Brad and Shelagh for their long-suffering tolerance and support over the last year while we have been glued to our laptops.

Janet Griffiths and Steve Boyle

Dedicated to

The residents of Royal Earlswood Hospital (Surrey), Greaves Hall Hospital (Merseyside), and Ely Hospital (Cardiff) who are now living in the community, to the people of Beira in Mozambique, and the many disabled people and their carers we have met personally and professionally, who are still fighting for equal rights; they are the inspiration for this guide.

HOLISTIC ORAL CARE –
a guide for health professionals

Contents

Introduction: How to use this guide

Section 1: Principles and practice of oral health care

This section of the guide forms the core knowledge and skills required by all health professionals and carers undertaking oral care. Many of the later, more specialised chapters refer back to this section, and so if you only read one section, this is the one to concentrate on first!

A description of the main oral diseases is followed by the basic principles and practice of oral care that a self-caring adult would be expected to carry out. For people in your care this is the level of care, which you should be aiming to achieve oral health. The two broad groups of children, and of the older person and their differing oral needs are then examined.

The section concludes with a chapter on dental services and the different types of dental teams. This chapter has been included in this section to enable the health professional to access effectively the most appropriate aspect of the service. As the organisation of oral health services at a primary care level is constantly evolving we recognise that the reader may find differing delivery systems in their locality.

After reading Section 1, look at the most appropriate section for your clients' needs. Most health care professionals will require criteria for assessing oral health needs. These are covered in the next section.

Section 2: A guide to oral assessment and oral health care

This is aimed primarily at the nurse providing care in a hospital or community setting. The guidelines, criteria and procedures are based on a wide variety of settings. This section should be used as a check list for the requirements to create an environment which is supportive of oral health, rather than the converse which often creates barriers to oral health.

The first chapter examines key indicators for oral health and reviews current assessment systems. The objective is to assist with the nursing process in formulating care plans based on meeting the individual's oral needs.

The suggested role of the manager in nursing and other care settings is outlined in the following chapter as the key person controlling resources and staff. Although identified as a manager, this key person may have a variety of roles. However, the principle underpinning this chapter is that one person should be delegated to oversee the development of oral care, keep it on the agenda, facilitate training and manage the required resources.

Chapter 8 summarises the major oral side-effects of medication and their potential impact on oral health. Later sections provide more specific detail on oral side-effects.

Section 2 closes with a review of the tools, equipment and materials needed to provide oral care. It is recognised that many clients will require varying degrees of assistance to meet their individual oral needs.

Now select the chapter most appropriate to your client group for an overview of their oral condition, the effects on oral health, and how oral care may need to be modified.

Section 3: At-risk groups: people with specific oral health needs

This section provides a comprehensive review of the commoner conditions and diseases and their possible impact on oral health, including medication and treatment. There have been considerable changes recently in the terminology associated with impairment, disability and handicap, so the first chapter reviews the development of terminology and refers to the requirements of the Disability Discrimination Act.

Chapter 11 addresses conditions that appear in childhood. Subsequent chapters take a systemic approach to conditions that generally appear in adult life. Although there will be inevitable exclusions and oversights, we believe that we have covered most modifying factors from the perspective of oral health.

Section 4: Oral health promotion

This section is designed to address the health promotion aspects of oral health care. This is a central theme of primary health care, with almost everyone being familiar with the maxim that prevention is better than cure. This section examines how oral health promotion can be more fully integrated into wider health promotion. It is now widely recognised that oral health issues should be considered in the wider promotion of health, this is known as the common risk approach. Emerging research is beginning to demonstrate a potential link between oral disease and other challenges to health. Although at first it may appear that this section is aimed at specialised health care workers with clearly identified roles in health promotion, we recognise that health promotion should form part of every health intervention. Even for the most dependent individual there is always some potential for health promotion and some way of maximising the potential for self care.

In Chapter 19 a widely accepted model of health promotion is used as a model of demonstrating how oral health can be considered within general health promotion.

Chapter 20 provides clear practical guidance for health promotion in different settings. The practice of health promotion has evolved over the years and we have included some examples of aims and objectives of actual programmes currently being delivered that conform to best practice in health promotion.

Finally, we hope that you will use this guide as part of your daily health care activities. It was not produced for a 'read-once-and-onto-the-shelf' approach!

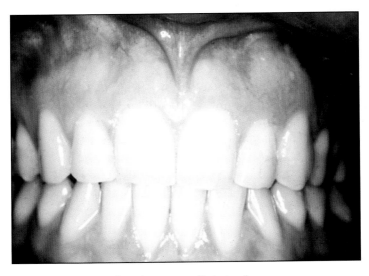

A healthy adult mouth - what we are all aiming for

Section 1: Principles and practice of oral health care

This section forms the central core knowledge that is required by all health professionals and carers involved in holistic oral care. The basic preventive methods of the commonest oral diseases and methods for maintaining oral health are described in Chapters 1 and 2. These two chapters are concerned with the self-caring adult and the principles of oral care they would follow. The differing needs of children and older people are examined in Chapters 3 and 4. The section concludes with a detailed examination of dental services and the dental team in the UK. We recognise that there will be differences across the devolved countries and it is likely that the effects of devolving commissioning of primary health care to a local level will be evident. The aim of this Chapter is to assist the health professional or carer to help those in their care to access the most appropriate service and member of the dental team.

Chapter 1

Oral health and disease

1.1 The 'World's Commonest Disease'

The 'World's Commonest Disease' is actually composed of two common diseases, periodontal (gum) disease and dental caries (tooth decay). It is largely self inflicted, although some individuals are not necessarily able to influence their own lifestyles and the societal factors to practice effective prevention. As the mouth acts as a 'mirror' of general health, there may also be oral manifestations of general diseases and conditions. In addition, there are rarer oral infections and more life-threatening oral cancers.

1.2 Periodontal disease

Although periodontal disease is the single largest cause of tooth loss in adults, with 50% of older people losing one or more teeth[1], the early signs and symptoms of periodontal disease, which are gums that bleed during

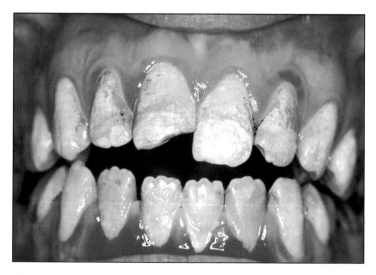

Figure 1.1 Severe gingivitis in a young male with learning difficulties. Areas of enamel opacity may have been caused by decayed primary teeth affecting the developing secondary dentition or may be related to neo-natal illness. The upper teeth show the neo-natal line and a blue tinge, which is suggestive of Tetracyeline staining

brushing, are often not recognised as abnormal *(Figure 1.1)*. Other, later signs of periodontal disease, such as receding gums and loose teeth, are still often seen as part of the ageing process by many people and health professionals *(Figure 1.2)*. Although 95% of the adult population will exhibit some effects of periodontal disease, the severity of disease varies enormously. It poses a higher threat to the dentition of approximately 10-15% of the population who are more susceptible to the damaging effects

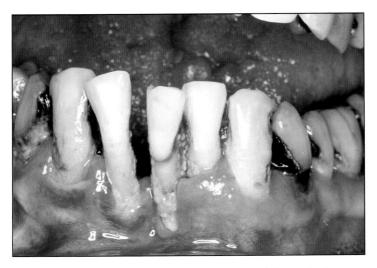

Figure 1.2 Gingival recession with chronic periodontal disease leading to mobility of the two lower central teeth. Calculus is visible on the roots

and 10% of the older population will lose the majority of their teeth[1].

Periodontal disease is a collective term for a number of conditions that affect the supporting fibres linking the teeth to the surrounding bone and the associated tissues covering them. *Figure 1.3* shows a diagrammatic cross-section of a healthy tooth. Periodontal diseases affect the gingiva, periodontal fibres and supporting bone shown on the diagram.

In lay terms, the 'gum' is a description of all the mucous membranes that cover the supporting bones and musculature of the jaws. In anatomical terms, there is a differentiation between the 'gingival tissue' which consists of the free and attached tissues over the bone in which are inserted the roots of the teeth, and the rest of the soft tissues in the mouth.

1.3 Chronic periodontitis

The commonest of the periodontal diseases is chronic periodontitis. This condition often begins in childhood with inflamed gum margins. The reddened, swollen gum margins bleed when brushed as they are more fragile than healthy gum tissue. This stage is referred to as 'gingivitis' and is usually controllable with more effective and regular toothbrushing *(Figure 1.1)*. The condition is reversible and no lasting damage to the gums should occur. However the condition can progress to 'chronic periodontitis' in which the fibres and bone supporting the teeth are affected *(Figure 1.2)*. This may progress to persistent infection, receding of

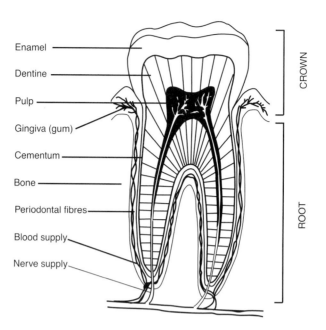

Enamel

Dentine

Pulp

Gingiva (gum)

Cementum

Bone

Periodontal fibres

Blood supply

Nerve supply

CROWN

ROOT

Figure 1.3 A diagrammatic cross-section of a healthy tooth

the gingival tissue exposing the roots of the teeth and loosening of the teeth. In the later stages the teeth may require extraction. Although virtually all adults exhibit some effects of chronic periodontitis, the rate at which the condition progresses varies enormously between individuals.

Causes and modifying factors

Periodontal disease is caused by 'dental plaque'. This is a descriptive term for the layer of bacteria on teeth which is present in all mouths. Plaque will build up on any surface in the mouth, whether natural or artificial, but only to any appreciable degree in those areas where it is not removed by the normal movements of speech and eating.

The normal anatomy of the teeth and gums creates a space in which plaque can accumulate, and a number of other factors can contribute to a potentially damaging build-up. These factors include malpositioned teeth, badly contoured fillings and some types of dentures. In some parts of the mouth, the formation of 'calculus' or 'tartar' will act as a rough surface on teeth, permitting a greater build-up of plaque *(Figures 1.2, 1.4, 1.5)*.

After a period of several days the colony of micro-organisms in the plaque will produce enough toxins and by-products to initiate a response from the tissues. This is the normal inflammatory response to any injury or

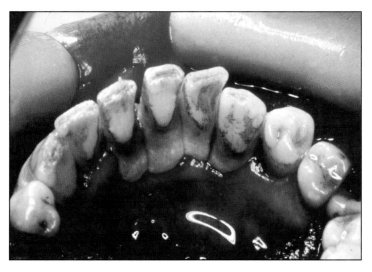

Figure 1.4 Calculus and staining behind the lower front teeth. This is an area prone to calculus because of its proximity to the sublingual salivary glands

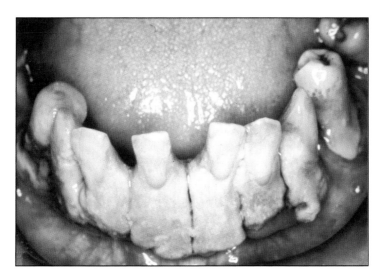

Figure 1.5 Very heavy deposits of calculus on the lower front teeth, evidence of poor oral hygiene and dental neglect

infection. If the irritant plaque is not removed, this response becomes chronic and progressive and there will be some tissue destruction and repair. Eventually the supporting bone and periodontal fibres are destroyed and replaced by fibrous tissue.

There are variations in the bacterial composition of dental plaque between individuals and even between different sites in the mouth. This may account for some of the differences seen in the rate at which disease progresses. Hormonal and metabolic changes during pregnancy and puberty, or linked to disorders such as diabetes, can also alter the response, but in many cases there is no identifiable reason. There is also considerable evidence that smoking will increase the risk of developing periodontal disease and compromise treatment[1]. As in all chronic infections, the response of the individual's immune system will alter the progress of the disease, and there is no reason to suggest that chronic periodontal disease should be an exception. Any chronic debilitating condition can affect the gums either directly or by impairing the individual's ability to maintain oral hygiene.

Prevention

The main approach to prevention is to control the formation and build-up of plaque. Even though it is not feasible to sterilise the mouth and rid it permanently of bacteria, plaque can be prevented from accumulating at sites in the mouth and reaching the stage of provoking an inflammatory condition. Plaque control depends on the individual being able to maintain effective oral hygiene. One of the main aims of this book is to enable individuals who are dependent to some extent on others for their daily needs to be effectively achieving this.

Summary of preventive methods for periodontal disease

Chapter 2 describes the basic principles of plaque control for the self-caring adult. These consist of:

- Daily removal of plaque from the gum margins
- Regular removal of calculus (tartar) by members of the dental team
- Regular dental attendance to monitor early signs of disease.

1.4 Dental caries

The main condition affecting the tooth itself is dental caries or dental decay (*Figures 1.6 – 1.8*). The tooth is composed of an outer layer of enamel, the hardest substance in the body. The second layer of dentine is also highly mineralised. The pulp chamber contains nerves and the blood supply that maintains the vitality of the tooth. Dental caries starts in the outer covering of enamel with a small area losing some of its mineral content. Once the enamel is breached, the process continues through the soft layer of dentine underneath. This can undermine the structure of the tooth and a cavity may form. The cavity, if untreated, will continue to enlarge until the living pulp is reached and direct infection will occur. The resulting infection can track

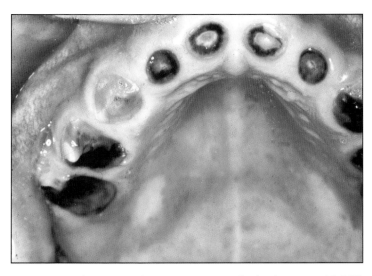

Figure 1.6 Bottle caries in the upper primary teeth of a three-year-old child

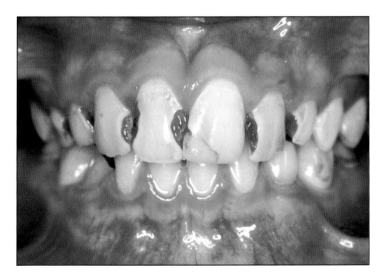

Figure 1.7 Advanced caries in the mixed dentition of a nine-year-old child. Cavities are easily visible between the four upper front teeth; these are the secondary teeth, which have only been present for a few years. The child had a dietary history of at least nine cans of carbonated drinks daily and never drank any other liquids

the length of the root canal and an abscess may form *(Figure1.9)*. The sequence of events can be summarised by the equation:

Plaque+Sugar → Acid+Tooth Surface → Dental Caries

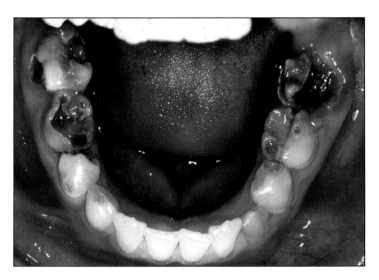

Figure 1.8 The lower jaw of the same case to that shown in Figure 1.7. The last visible decayed tooth is the first permanent molar tooth, which appears around six years of age

Signs and symptoms of dental caries

Healthy enamel and dentine form an effective insulation for the nerve fibres in the pulp chamber and a healthy tooth will not react to changes in temperature unless they are excessive. The sensitivity experienced by some people is often due to the transmission of temperature changes from an exposed root area to the nerve. This is a sequel of gum disease and associated recession of the gum margin.

In the earlier stages of dental decay, the tooth may be painful only in the transmission of hot and cold, which is due to the loss of insulating enamel and dentine. The symptoms and signs of the later stages are obvious to the individual, with severe pain and swelling as the contents of the pulp chamber become inflamed.

It may take up to several years for significant damage in the form of a large cavity, visible to the naked eye, to develop and the early stages may be completely symptom-free and painless.

Dental decay can also attack the roots of the teeth if they are exposed following recession in gum disease. This is more often seen in older people and is also seen in association with certain forms of drug abuse.

Cause of dental caries

There is normally a balance at the surface of the tooth between mineral on the surface of the enamel leaving the tooth, being held in suspension in saliva and then being laid back down again. This balance will be disturbed by the presence of acids. If the pH reduces from a neutral 7 to below 5.5 there will be a net loss of mineral. At this stage dental caries begins. The acid derives from the bacteria present in dental plaque, as a by-product of their metabolic processes. The bacteria break down certain dietary sugars, particularly sucrose, for energy and growth. As this happens the plaque colony will grow and help to retain the acid in contact with the tooth, and promote further demineralisation.

Factors affecting dental decay

The single largest factor in promoting dental caries is the number of times that sugars are consumed. It takes just a couple of minutes for the bacteria in plaque to produce enough acid to tip the mineral balance towards a net loss of mineral. This imbalance (sometimes known as an 'acid attack')

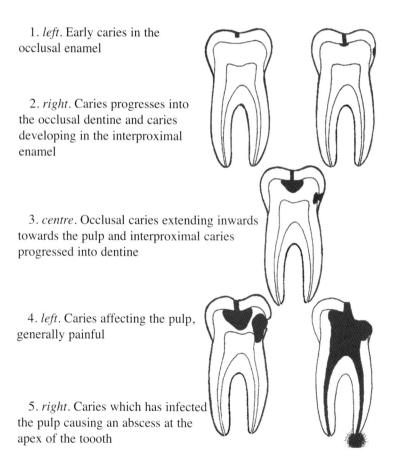

1. *left*. Early caries in the occlusal enamel

2. *right*. Caries progresses into the occlusal dentine and caries developing in the interproximal enamel

3. *centre*. Occlusal caries extending inwards towards the pulp and interproximal caries progressed into dentine

4. *left*. Caries affecting the pulp, generally painful

5. *right*. Caries which has infected the pulp causing an abscess at the apex of the toooth

Figure 1.9 The decay process. The resulting infection can track the length of the root canal and an abscess may form

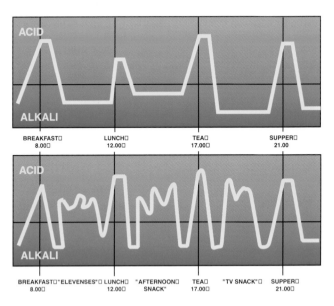

Figure 1.10 The effects of frequent consumption of sugar and the extended periods during which the oral environment is acidic

takes up to an hour to neutralise. Another ingestion of sugar during that period will prolong the time during which the mouth is acidic and therefore promotes dental caries. *Figure 1.10* shows the effects of frequent consumption of sugar and the extended periods during which the oral environment is acidic.

Saliva can help to neutralise the acids produced by plaque bacteria. There is a reduction in the normal salivary flow at night and this creates even more favourable conditions for plaque to proliferate. In later chapters the effects of some medication on saliva flow will be highlighted as leaving individuals more susceptible to dental caries.

The resistance of the tooth to dental caries appears to vary between individuals, although the significance of this factor is difficult to calculate or predict. The process of dental caries is an extremely complex one to describe in lay terms and often the explanation of natural resistance has been erroneously used. It should be used with caution as it implies that there is little in personal behaviour that can be done to control and prevent further dental decay.

Besides reducing the frequency and quantity of sugars in the diet, the other important factor in preventing dental caries is fluoride. The most important effect of fluoride is to prevent the loss of calcium and phosphate ions at the surface of the tooth. To be most effective it should be used on a daily basis, either in drinking water, toothpaste or in daily supplements. Chapters 2 and 3 provide more detailed information on the use of fluoride.

No other supplements, such as calcium, have been shown to have any preventive effect on teeth. Similarly, malnutrition or dietary deficiencies during pregnancy have little effect on infants' teeth, except in very rare cases. Once calcium has been laid down in the tooth during development, only the decay process can remove it, there is no mechanism for a foetus to remove mineral from a mothers teeth during pregnancy as is often encountered in folklore and lay beliefs.

The role of tooth brushing in preventing dental decay

Tooth brushing alone will not prevent dental caries. The sites in the mouth where dental caries begins are very difficult, if not impossible, to render plaque free with a toothbrush. These sites are the pits and fissures of the chewing surfaces of the molars (occlusal surfaces) (*Figure 1.8*) and in between the teeth (interproximal surfaces) (*Figure 1.7*). Tooth brushing does have a role in removing plaque from the smooth surfaces of the enamel and as a method of applying fluoride toothpaste. As a plaque removal tool it is also the main preventive tool for gum disease.

Other methods of plaque control

Whilst it is impossible to eliminate plaque on a practical level, and indeed not even completely necessary, there are antiseptic agents which can inhibit its growth. These agents may be a useful aid to oral hygiene and Chapter 9 describes their appropriate use.

Eating fibrous foods like carrots and apples does not have any demonstrable effect on plaque levels, but they are certainly preferable to sweets as a healthy snack.

Summary of preventive methods for dental caries

Chapter 2 describes in detail the methods for prevention of dental caries for the self-caring adult. These consist of:

- Reducing the consumption, particularly the number of intakes, of sugar containing food and drinks
- Cleaning the teeth and gums every day with fluoride toothpaste
- Regular dental attendance for detection of early problems.

1.5 Oral Infections

Following periodontal diseases and dental caries there are a range of other oral infections. The next commonest infective organism is Candida which is often a marker of an underlying systemic condition. A range of viral infections from the Herpes virus can also have oral manifestations. (See Chapters 15 and 16).

1.6 Role of saliva in oral health

The role of saliva is crucial in maintaining oral health. Its functions are:

- Lubrication of the soft tissues
- Mechanical flushing of food and debris
- Neutralisation of acids caused by plaque and sugars
- Neutralisation of acids from acidic drinks and regurgitated stomach acids
- Providing minerals to strengthen the tooth surface
- Anti-bacterial effect.

These properties have obvious benefits in speech, mastication and swallowing, and in maintaining the health of both hard and soft tissues. The effects of reduced saliva flow in relation to specific conditions are highlighted in later chapters.

1.7 Oral cancer

Oral cancer is the most life-threatening of all oral diseases and is the eighth most common cancer in the UK[2]. Although there have been changes in the numbers of cases in different parts of the mouth and oral cavity, intra-oral cancers are increasing in the young adult[3].

Unfortunately, many cases are only diagnosed at an advanced stage as the early stages are frequently symptom-free (*Figures 1.11-1.13*). A late diagnosis has adverse effects on the patient's prognosis and life expectancy. Prevention, reducing risk factors and early detection are vitally important.

Risk factors for oral cancer

Depending on the site of the oral cancer, there are a number of associated risk factors:

Sunlight

Exposure to sunlight has been identified as a factor in cancer of the lip, with a high incidence in Caucasian people[4]. The lower incidence of lip

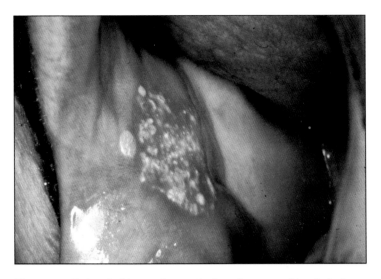

Figure 1.11 Red and white patches on the buccal mucosa; this relatively innocuous looking lesion is malignant

cancer amongst women has been attributed to the use of cosmetics[5] while the use of lip protection and sunscreen is advised for fair skinned people in sunnier climates[4].

Tobacco

Tobacco, whether smoked, chewed or taken as a snuff, is reported to be an important factor in the aetiology of oral cancer[6]. There is a strong relationship between cigarette smoking and cancer of the mouth[6]. Pipe smoking is linked with cancer of the lip which may be partly due to the excessive heat generated producing a chronic irritation of the tissues[6]. The practice of reverse smoking, with the lit end in the mouth, is common in some Asian communities and countries and is associated with cancer of the hard palate. The use of snuff and other smokeless uses of tobacco such as betel quid chewing, tobacco pouches and Pan chewing has also been strongly implicated in the rise of oral cancers[7].

Alcohol

High alcohol consumption is implicated in the aetiology of oral cancer. Certain occupations with easy access to alcohol show a higher incidence in comparison to groups that abstain[8]. The risk is significantly increased when alcohol is consumed with tobacco[8]. The rise in consumption patterns of alcohol and cigarette smoking in women is linked with the rising proportion of female cases of oral cancer. Although tobacco usage has reduced in many industrialised countries[8] there has not been a reduction in oral cancers. This suggests that high alcohol consumption is becoming more important as a risk factor[9].

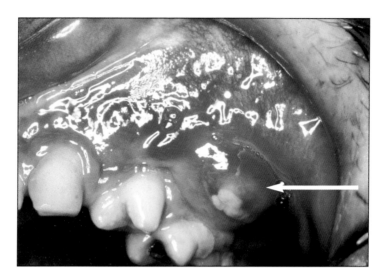

Figure 1.12 Carcinoma of the maxilla

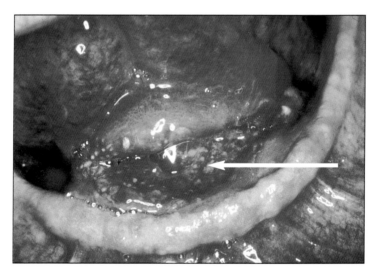

Figure 1.13 Carcinoma of the floor of the mouth; the patient complained of soreness caused by dentures and an ulcer that would not heal

Dental factors

Although it seems that local factors, for example, poor oral hygiene and local irritations due to poorly fitting dentures, may be risk factors, it is hard to demonstrate clear research[9] to support this.

Nutritional factors, infections and viruses

Nutritional deficiencies may increase susceptibility to oral cancer as well as to certain lesions of the mucous membrane, which become infected by candida organisms. Viral infections, in particular herpes simplex, human papilloviruses and fungal infections are also under suspicion[4]. However antioxidants, common in fruit and vegetables may have a preventive effect[1].

One of the roles for those involved in oral care is early detection of pre-malignant and malignant stages as early diagnosis is so important to the outcome of treatment. Later sections illustrate some of the conditions that could arouse suspicion. Regular annual oral screening is an important process to aid early diagnosis[4].

1.8 Distribution of oral disease

Dental caries

Over the centuries, there have been several changes in the rate of dental caries that have closely mirrored changing patterns of sugar consumption. *Figure 1.14* shows the dramatic increase that occurred from the 17th century onwards once imported cane sugar became more widely available[10].

Changes in technique for milling flour produced a more refined product

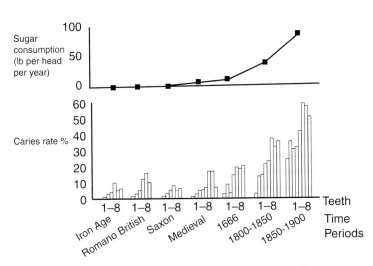

Figure 1.14 Historical sugar consumption and caries rates in the permanent dentitions of British populations. Reproduced from Dental Update by kind permission of George Warman Publications (UK) Ltd

which was less abrasive to teeth and did not eradicate the fissures of the occlusal surfaces where much decay starts. Further increases were seen due to the import of wheat products that substantially changed eating patterns. In other communities, for example the Inuit community, there was not even a word in their language for toothache until the introduction of sugar candy in their diet following contact with the USA culture[11].

Sugar consumption rose during the 19th century with the removal of tariffs; this rise was only temporarily halted by sugar rationing in both World Wars. These temporary declines in sugar consumption were also accompanied by temporary reductions in dental caries.

Although sugar consumption has been fairly constant at an average of 40kg per person per year for the last few decades[12], there has been a dramatic reduction in the amount of dental caries in industrialised countries.

The main reasons for the fall in dental caries are:

- Wider use of fluoride containing toothpastes
- Greater awareness of the importance of good dental health
- Increased availability of dental resources
- A more preventive approach to dental care, particularly the use of fissure sealants.

Although the total consumption of sugar remains high with the UK population consuming the most confectionery in Europe, there have been changes in patterns of consumption in social and cultural groups[13]. Dental caries is very much a social deprivation related condition and it still remains a substantial health problem. When examined in more detail, there is a demonstrable gradient[14] in the dental decay experience across parts of the UK. Within districts, it can be seen that many of the factors associated with social deprivation and poverty are also linked with high decay rates. Apparent racial differences are mainly due to social deprivation, including language barriers[7]. In developing countries there has been an increase in dental decay experience that is particularly marked in urban populations[13] that have greater access to more refined sugar products.

Periodontal disease

The distribution and trends in periodontal disease are more difficult to define as there are different criteria for measuring the disease. It is still relatively difficult to identify the section of the population at high risk of developing progressively destructive periodontal disease. Data at the WHO Global Bank demonstrate that the signs of poor oral hygiene,

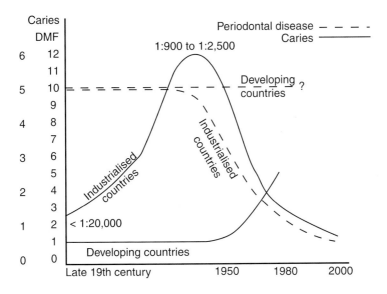

Figure 1.15 Projections of future trends in the percentage of UK adults without natural teeth, 1998-2028. Reproduced from Dental Update by kind permission of George Warman Publications (UK) Ltd

bleeding gums and calculus, are decreasing in industrialised societies. In developing countries, oral hygiene is generally poorer and there are scarcer dental resources. *Figure 1.15* summarises the current oral health trends for the last century[10].

Tooth loss

The avoidance of tooth loss is the primary goal of dental health, and there have been major changes over the recent decades. The latest UK Adult Health Survey showed a continued reduction in tooth loss, *Figure 1.16* showing the trend over the last 30 years[15]. It is expected that by 2028 only 4% of the adult population will be edentulous.

1.9 General impairment and oral handicap

In addition to the influences of a person's environment, values and beliefs and the presence of any general impairment may produce or worsen an oral handicap. The OPCS survey of disability[16], examined its prevalence in Britain and looked at it in terms of the functional effects upon daily living. The functions identified included:

- Locomotion
- Dexterity

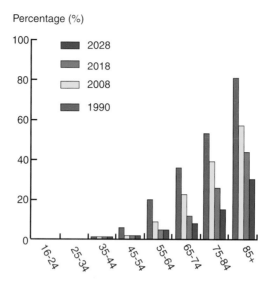

Percentage (%)

Figure 1.16 Projections of future trends in the percentage of UK adults without natural teeth, 1998-2028. Reproduced by kind permission of the author and the Editor of the British Dental Journal

- Hearing
- Continence
- Behaviour
- Reaching and stretching
- Seeing
- Personal care
- Communication
- Intellectual functioning.

For most of these functions, disability will restrict or prevent a person carrying out the aspects of normal care necessary to maintain oral health. The extent to which disability may contribute to oral handicap is considerable with over six million adults above the threshold level of disability. Members of the health care team and carers need to be aware of the implications of disability in contributing to oral handicap. Later sections will deal with disability from a functional viewpoint.

1.10 Demographic changes and oral health

The UK population is ageing. The proportion of older people has increased and is projected to rise. As lifespan is also increasing the proportion of old and very old people will also grow dramatically. It is predicted that there will be significantly more older people in the population who will need dental care and who will present with a broad range of dependent conditions. There will be a broadening gap in the amount of disposable income with a significant proportion of older people being able to fund their own dental care, although many will also rely on public services. As a lot of impairing conditions are age related there will be different challenges for the dental team.

1.11 Prevention of oral disease and oral ill health

There are a number of processes in which partnership working is essential between the dental team and other health care teams.

Primary prevention

This is prevention before the appearance of disease and includes promoting positive health. In oral health, this involves:

- Establishing a well balanced diet in which sugars form a low proportion
- A reduction from the average 40kg of sugar consumption to 10-15kg per year
- Effective oral hygiene
- Use of fluoride containing toothpaste
- Regular dental attendance
- Encouraging positive values and self reliance in oral health
- Smoking and alcohol counselling.

The role of all members of the dental team is very evident when incorporating oral health into a holistic approach to good health.

Secondary prevention

As oral diseases are extremely prevalent there may be some failure in the primary preventive process. However the value of establishing and reinforcing preventive regimes can help to minimise further disease and reduce an oral handicap. The presence of existing disease can be a strong motivator to initiate more effective preventive approaches to avoid future disease. It is a common health belief for people not to regard themselves susceptible to disease even though there may be predisposing factors in their lifestyle or environment.

1.12 Summary

Oral and dental disease consists of a number of conditions. The most important can be categorised as follows:

- Dental caries (dental decay) (*Figures 1.6 – 1.8*)
- Periodontal disease (gum disease) (*Figures 1.1 and 1.2*)
- Oral infections (*Figures 2.5, 2.6, 15.1 - 15.3, 16.1*)
- Oral cancers (*Figures 1.11 – 1.13*)

Although dental caries and periodontal disease are caused by oral bacteria in dental plaque, there are many factors which will dictate how much an individual is predisposed to the conditions.
These factors include:

- Social, cultural and economic
- Sugar consumption
- Oral hygiene
- Access to dental services
- Use of tobacco
- Alcohol consumption
- Local dental factors.

An effective preventive strategy will involve the whole dental team working in partnership with all agencies concerned with health.

References

1. Levine R, Stillman-Lowe C. The scientific basis of oral health education. 5th Edition. London: British Dental Association, 2004.
2. Parkin D, Pisani M, Ferlay J. Estimates of world-wide incidence of eighteen major cancers in 1985. *Int J Cancer* 1993 **54**: 594-606.
3. Johnson NW, Warnakulasuriya KAAS. Epidemiology and aetiology of oral cancer in the United Kingdom. *Community Dent Health* 1993 **10**: 13-29.
4. Johnson NW, Warnakulasuriya KAAS, Partridge M *et al.* Oral cancer- a serious and growing problem. *Ann R Coll Surg Eng* 1995 **77**: 321-322.
5. Binnie WH, Rankin KV. Epidemiology of oral cancer. In: *Oral cancer: clinical and pathological considerations.* pp 2-11. Florida: CRC Press, 1988.
6. Ogden GR, Macluskey M. An overview of the prevention of oral cancer and diagnostic markers of malignant change: 1. Prevention. *Dent Update* 2000 27: 95-99.

7. Dhawan N, Bedi R. Transcultural oral health care: 6. The oral health of minority ethnic groups in the United Kingdom. A review. *Dent Update* 2001 **28:** 30-34.

8. Hindle I, Downer MC, Moles DR *et al.* Is alcohol responsible for more intra-oral cancer? *Oral Oncology* 2000 **36:** 328-333.

9. Smith CJ. Oral cancer and precancer: background, epidemiology and aetiology. *Br Dent J* 1989 **167:** 377-383.

10. Renson CE. Global changes in carie prevalence and dental manpower requirements 3. The effect of manpower needs. Dental Update 1989 16:382-389.

11. Bang G, Kristoffersen T. Dental caries and diet in an Alaskan Eskimo population. *Scand J Dent Res* 1972 **80:** 440-444.

12. Dietary Sugars and Human Disease. 37. Committee on Medical Aspects of Food Policy. 1989, London. HMSO.

13. Joint WHO/FAO Expert consultation on diet, nutrition and the prevention of chronic diseases (2002: Geneva, Switzerland). Pp105-128.WHO Technical Report Series 916. 2003 World Health Organisation.

14. Murray J. Prevalence of dental caries: retrospect and prospect. *Dent Update* 1998 **25:** 374-378. *Br Dent J 2000* **189:** 598-603.

15. Steele JG, Treasure E, Pitts NB *et al.* Total tooth loss in the UK in 1998 and implications for the future. *Br Dent J 2000* **189:** 598-603.

16. Martin J., Meltzer H, Elliot D. The prevalence of disability among adults: Report 1. 1988. London, OPCS; Social Survey Division, HMSO.

Chapter 2

Basic principles and practice of oral care

2

2.1 Introduction

The aim of this chapter is to set out the basic core principles and practices for oral care. A thorough grasp of the knowledge and skills in this section will enable any of the modifications described in later sections to be applied to the individual, in particular those with a specific health care need.

As a starting point for the techniques necessary to maintain good oral health, the focus will be on the self-caring adult. For the average adult there are three basic requirements or social goals. These are:

> • **A functional set of teeth**
> • **A pleasing appearance**
> • **Freedom from pain and discomfort.**

To achieve and maintain these goals, the individual requires:

> • **A core of knowledge and health skills**
> • **Motivation**
> • **Access to the correct equipment and facilities**
> • **Opportunity and environment to put them into practice.**

The basic knowledge and skills for oral care encompass five areas:

> • **Tooth care**
> • **Gum care**
> • **Mouth tissue care**
> • **Care of dentures and appliances (prostheses)**
> • **Use of the dental team.**

2.2 Tooth care

As outlined earlier, a number of factors are required for dental caries to occur. A useful summary of the process in equation form is:

> **Plaque + Sugar → Acid + Tooth Surface → Dental Caries**

Prevention of dental decay requires steps to be taken at all stages of the equation:

• **Control and reduction of refined sugars in the diet**

• Effective plaque removal from tooth surfaces
• Strengthening the tooth surface.

2.3 Dietary care by reduction of refined sugars

The COMA report on 'Dietary Sugars and Human Disease' reviewed the evidence in depth[1], and the British Dental Association supports the evidence of the COMA report on the prevention of decay. A major report issued by the WHO/FAO also confirms the extent of evidence linking sugar consumption with dental decay[2] *(Table 2.1)*.

Table 2.1 Summary of strength of evidence linking diet to dental caries

Evidence	Decreased Risk	No relationship	Increased Risk
Convincing	Fluoride	Starch excluding cakes, biscuits, and snacks with added sugar	Amount of free sugars Frequency of sugars
Probable	Hard cheese Sugar-free chewing gum	Whole fresh fruit	
Possible	Xylitol Milk Dietary fibre		Undernutrition
Insufficient	Whole fresh fruit		Dried nuts

But even with clear evidence and straightforward processes the level of dental decay remains a major health problem. There are many factors to explain why averages of 40kg of refined sugars are consumed per person each year in the UK. Sugar containing food and drinks are used as part of many festivals, anniversaries and celebrations. They are used to console, reward, bribe and demonstrate affection. Sugar is also used extensively as a preservative and a bulking agent by the food industry. The patterns of how sugars are consumed have changed considerably over the last decades. Instead of being added as table sugar they are now consumed as part of prepared and manufactured foods. The frequency and time when sugars are consumed are also factors in their cariogenicity. *Figure1.10* demonstrates how frequent consumption of sugars between mealtimes will keep the oral environment acidic and promote caries.

One important factor is powerful and intensely persuasive advertising backed by huge budgets to promote products. However there now exist many strategies for reducing and replacing sugars in the diet with non-cariogenic sweeteners. Many people also aim to reduce consumption of sugars as part of calorie-controlled diets.

A range of cariogenic sugars

The COMA report did not define sugars in terms of their origin or level of refinement but in their degree of availability to plaque bacteria. This divides sugars into two broad groups, those intrinsic to cell walls and those extrinsic to cell walls.

Intrinsic sugars

These form an integral part of unprocessed foods, mainly fruit and vegetables. Even though these sugars are mainly fructose, glucose and sucrose, they are not an available source of energy to plaque bacteria in the oral environment and therefore are a negligible cause of dental caries.

Extrinsic sugars

These are not located within the cellular structure of food. They fall into two groups.

- Milk sugars: which occur naturally in milk and milk products. They are almost entirely lactose and are a negligible cause of dental decay except under certain circumstances.
- Non-milk extrinsic sugars (NME): which include 'added sugars' from recipe and table sugars, and honey.

This last group, with the most unwieldy name is often known colloquially by health educators as NME or 'enemy' sugars! For those with the scientific training to decipher food labelling, it is evident that many refined foods have added sucrose. This includes many snack foods, even those that are savoury. By design they are intended to be consumed between meals in small portions which increases the number of times that the oral environment is below pH 5.5 and demineralisation can occur.

2.4 Prevention of dental caries

The first step in a plan to reduce the consumption of refined sugars is to identify the frequency and quantity in the diet. A diet sheet (*Figure 2.1*) can be a useful tool. The next step is to advise a gradual substitution to less damaging alternatives with a particular focus on snack food and drinks. As a general principle sugars should form no more than 10% of the daily diet. An holistic approach to healthy eating should be promoted, encouraging a diet that is low in saturated fat and salt, high in fibre and contains the recommended daily amounts of fruit and vegetables (*Table 2.2*).

Time	Food/Drink	Quantity	Eaten where	Doing
Day 1				
Day 2				
Day 3				

Figure 2.1 An example of a diet sheet

2.5 Plaque control and the prevention of dental caries

The dental caries equation described earlier included the presence of dental plaque. The bacteria in dental plaque utilise the dietary sugars and the metabolic process lowers the pH of the oral environment and promotes demineralisation.

Examination of many people's mouths shows that dental decay has occurred in two main sites: the occlusal surfaces of molar teeth and the interproximal areas (*Figures 1.7, 1.8* and *2.2*). These are the areas from which it is most difficult to remove plaque efficiently. It is difficult, if not impossible to manipulate a toothbrush into the depths of the fissures of the occlusal surface. In addition, the process of demineralisation takes place within two minutes of consuming a caries-mediating sugar. This considerably decreases the chance of plaque being removed before damage can occur.

Table 2.2 The five food groups[3]

	Examples	**Message**
Bread, cereals and potatoes	Breakfast cereals, rice, oats, noodles, maize, millet, yams, plantain, beans, pulses	Eat lots
Fruit and vegetables	Fresh, frozen and canned fruit, vegetables and dried fruit. A glass of fruit juice, beans and pulses	Eat five portions a day. Fruit juice only counts as one portion, beans and pulses only count as one portion
Milk and dairy foods	Milk, cheese, yoghurt, fromage frais. Not butter, eggs and cream	Eat or drink moderate amounts and choose low fat versions
Meat, fish and alternatives	Meat, poultry, fish, eggs, nuts. Beans and pulses for vegetarians. Fish includes frozen, canned. Aim to eat at least one portion of oily fish each week	Eat or drink moderate amounts and choose low fat versions
Food containing fat: foods and drinks containing sugar	Foods containing fat: Margarine, butter, other spreading fats, cooking oils Foods containing sugar: Soft drinks, sweets, cakes, pudding, ice cream	Eat sparingly and look for low fat alternatives Foods and drinks containing sugar should be eaten mainly at mealtimes to reduce the risk of dental caries

It is important to practise good plaque control by brushing the teeth to remove all plaque and debris from the smooth surfaces and gum margins in order to prevent decay of these surfaces. However, there are other aids to plaque control besides a toothbrush. These include dental floss or tape, woodsticks and interdental brushes. As a general principle, people should be taught individually by a member of the clinical dental team how to use these effectively.

There are several types of mouthwashes that claim to improve plaque control. The only products with proven clinical benefit are those

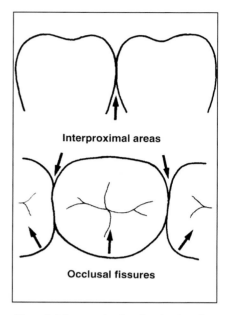

Figure 2.2 Interproximal and occlusal surfaces

containing chlorhexidine[4]. In the format of mouthwashes, gels and sprays, products containing chlorhexidine have a valuable role in the control of gum disease.

2.6 Fluoride products

Measures that strengthen the tooth's enamel can help create a surface that is more resistant to attack by acids. For the average self-caring adult, this involves the application of fluoride containing products directly to the surfaces of the teeth.

The simplest, cheapest and most common method is by brushing with fluoride-containing toothpaste. The widespread use of these toothpastes has been one of the major factors in the large reduction of dental decay in children[5].

Fluoride supplements in the form of daily or weekly rinses can be self-administered[6]. Fluoride, as a gel, is usually applied by a member of the dental team, although there are products available for home use which are also effective[7]. Fluoride supplements in the form of daily tablets or drops can produce significant reductions in dental decay in both the primary and secondary dentition *(Table 2.3)*. The benefits are greatest when the supplements are used regularly and with certain high-risk groups[8]. The benefits of fluoride arise from the regular topical effects and also by being incorporated into the developing tooth structure.

Table 2.3. Daily dosage for fluoride supplements for children in areas with less than 0.3ppm F in the water supply

6 months to 3 years	0.25mg F (0.5mg NaF)
3 years up to 6 years	0.5mg F (1.1mg NaF)
6 years and over	1.0mg F (2.2mg NaF)

The most effective method of fluoride supplementation is by adjusting the level of fluoride in the drinking water to one part per million. This is currently only available to approximately 10% of the UK population, in the West Midlands and the North East. This is in comparison with the USA where over 60% of the cities use fluoridated water. There are clear reductions in the levels of dental caries of the children in those areas in comparison with comparable areas[9].The greatest benefits are seen in children and in social classes IV and V who can experience up to five times more dental decay.

Progress in the extension of fluoridation of public water supplies has been slow. Nearly half the previous health authorities in England have requested their water companies to fluoridate the water supply[10] although the current legislation (The Water (Fluoridation) Act 1985) did not oblige the water companies to comply. Doubts about the safety of the procedure have been extensively examined by a systematic review[9]. The review found that fluoridating water helps to reduce tooth decay, with no clear evidence of potential adverse effects, other than the slight risk of mottling of the teeth. A new clause to the Act allowing targeted water fluoridation following consultation led by health authorities was passed in 2003 which should result in new schemes. A recent amendment to the Water Act in 2004 obliges water suppliers to fluoridate water supplies when directed to by a Strategic Health Authority in England or the Welsh Assembly Government.

2.7 Dietary control of acids

Frequent exposure of the tooth enamel to acids in the oral environment can lead to a generalised loss, dental erosion. The sources of the acids include:
  • Stomach acid regurgitation from gastric illness, anorexia or bulimia (*Figure 2.3*)

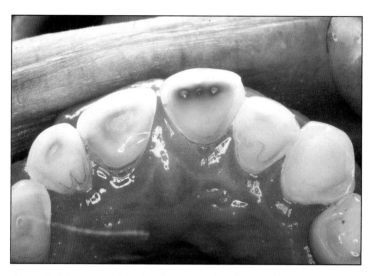

Figure 2.3 Erosion of the palatal surfaces of teeth caused by persistent acid regurgitation

- Foods with a high acid content including lemons, vinegar, pickles, fruit juices
- Drinks, including some carbonated drinks and sports drinks
- Some occupations which expose the workforce to acid aerosols including some chemical industries, although this is now reduced due to Health and Safety improvements.

A careful analysis of the diet can identify a dietary cause. The drinking of acidic drinks through a straw will reduce enamel exposure. Changes in the diet, advice on correct tooth brushing techniques and topically applied fluoride are the most effective methods of limiting further damage. In severe cases the professional application of fluoride under soft splints may be required. It is also important to be aware of the high acidic content of some medications including Vitamin C supplements, iron tonics and acid replacement therapy.

2.8 Gum care

The major cause of tooth loss for adults is gum disease, chronic destructive periodontitis. The most effective method of prevention is daily, thorough removal of dental plaque from the gum margins by brushing[8].

A self-caring adult can most effectively remove plaque using a systematic approach with a toothbrush and toothpaste. There are many different tooth

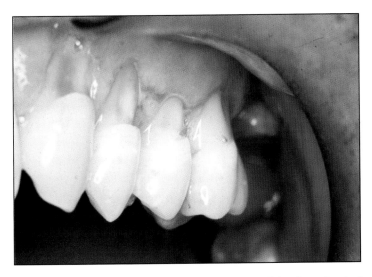

Figure 2.4 Abrasion caused by excessive horizontal tooth brushing, 'sawing' into the weaker dentine at the gum margin

brushing techniques, but one of the most effective is the simplest using short scrubbing or rotary movements. The use of a vigorous 'sawing' technique with a horizontal movement can cause harmful abrasion. This approach can create grooves in the necks of the teeth that may require restorations (*Figure 2.4*).

Similarly, there are many types of toothbrush available. The general guidelines are to select a small to medium headed brush with dense nylon filaments of a medium texture. The brush will need replacing when the filaments become 'splayed'. A variety of different heads may be advised for awkward areas. The shape of the handle appears to be immaterial providing all surfaces of the teeth can be reached including the buccal, palatal and lingual. The compromise of a fairly straight handle is often the most effective.

There is also a large range of electric toothbrushes available. There is some evidence to show that some models can be more effective in plaque removal[11]. Most have a small brush head that can aid access and they are certainly useful for people who have problems manipulating a manual toothbrush.

There are few guidelines for the selection of toothpaste. Providing the product contains fluoride the choice rests on individual taste, price and brand loyalty[12]. There are a variety of claims from manufacturers as to the efficacy of their products. Some of the stain removing toothpastes are very abrasive and should only be used occasionally. The desensitising ranges of toothpastes appear to have some benefit in reducing painful sensations in sensitive exposed dentine.

Many people have an inefficient brushing technique and plaque can accumulate around gum margins. As these margins become inflamed and more friable they are more likely to bleed when brushed. This is a very common finding, so most people do not even recognise it as a sign of disease. Healthy gums will not bleed following normal brushing and this provides an effective indicator of an individual's brushing. Even inflamed gums will respond to thorough brushing and return to a healthy condition following regular, effective brushing for a few days. *Figure 1.1* shows the appearance of gingivitis, the chronic inflammation of the gum margin. Dental plaque is difficult to detect in the early stages and the use of a vegetable dye in disclosing tablets or solutions can be useful *(Figure 9.2)*.

As well as regular brushing, the use of dental floss or woodsticks may be advised to clean the interproximal areas. These will also improve plaque removal from around the margins of crowns and bridgework. Individual advice from a dental clinician should be given on the use of these appliances.

The self-caring adult may occasionally need temporary help with plaque control provided by chlorhexidine containing products. This usually forms part of an active course of dental treatment. Long term use of these products can cause a surface staining of the teeth, but this can be removed by professional cleaning.

2.9 Mouth care

The only other regular care required by a self-caring adult for oral tissues is a gentle sweeping action of the buccal surfaces, tongue and palate. This should be accompanied by vigorous rinsing to remove retained food particles. Any tissues normally covered by dentures or other removable oral appliances should be rinsed with plain water. Antiseptic mouthwashes and gargles only give a short-term sensation of cleanliness and there is little evidence to show they have any benefits[4].

2.10 Malignant disease

It is worth considering other behaviours known to affect oral health. The use of tobacco is the highest risk in this category. The combination of both tobacco and high alcohol use greatly increases the risk of oral cancer[13]. The chewing of betel nut products and Quat has also been implicated in oral malignancy[14].

There is an increasing role for the dental team in assisting people to reduce and give up smoking[15]. As part of the clinical examination and history taking, routine questioning about smoking and offering support and information should be included.

2.11 Care of appliances

The types of oral appliances that the self-caring adult may wear fall into two main groups: removable and fixed. All appliances collect plaque and food debris.

Fixed appliances

These are semi-permanently or permanently attached to the teeth. By definition they must be cleaned in the mouth. They usually require individual tuition. Fluoride mouthwashes and chemical plaque control may be advised as added preventive measures. Fixed appliances include:

- Bridges to replace missing teeth
- Fixed Orthodontic appliances
- Wiring following jaw fractures or maxillofacial surgery.

Bridges

The same general principles apply to the care of bridges as natural teeth. This includes tooth brushing and the use of dental floss. Disclosing solutions used occasionally can be useful to highlight areas of plaque accumulation.

Orthodontic appliances

A fixed orthodontic appliance may carry complex wires and springs attached to brackets bonded to teeth. It will require very thorough cleaning with a soft toothbrush and individual instruction is recommended.

Wiring

Caring for the mouth which has been immobilised by wires and splints following fracture or surgery poses obvious problems for the efficient removal of plaque and debris. Even though the person may be nourished by a liquid or semi-liquid diet, they will still be at risk from dental decay. The difficulty of maintaining healthy gums will also increase the level of oral discomfort. In addition to tooth brushing, chlorhexidine mouthwash or spray may be also used to supplement plaque control.

Removable appliances

These can be removed for thorough cleaning and include:

- Full dentures
- Partial dentures
- Removable orthodontic appliances
- Obturators
- Other prostheses replacing hard and soft tissues.

Dentures

Even though there have been considerable improvements in oral health, there still remains a high percentage of older people who are denture wearers[16.] Dentures should be removed after eating and rinsed clean. Daily cleaning should be done over a bowl of water to prevent breakage if dropped. A soft brush and ordinary unperfumed soap followed by thorough rinsing will be sufficient in most cases. The following section contains more detailed advice. Partial dentures and appliances with wires and clasps are more prone to collect food and need more attention. The supporting teeth next to partial dentures also require additional attention. Calculus deposits and staining from food and tobacco may require cleaning in the dental surgery or laboratory. Poor denture hygiene is often associated with oral candida infections.

Removable orthodontic appliances

These should be cleaned carefully so as not to distort or damage the wires and springs. Unlike dentures, orthodontic appliances may be required to be worn at night. As saliva flow is reduced during the night, a high standard of oral care is necessary to avoid an increased risk of dental caries.

Obturators and facial prostheses

These appliances are individually constructed to close cleft palates or replace missing hard and soft tissues following maxillofacial surgery. They require the same basic care as dentures but any specific professional advice should be followed.

2.12 Denture care

Denture basics

Generally, all dentures should be left out of the mouth at night. Prolonged and repeated night use, particularly if the dentures are not plaque free, may lead to oral infections. The most common oral infection is oral candida (*Figures 2.5 and 2.6*). These infections are frequently unnoticed until they become acute. If dentures are worn frequently at night the wearer will need to maintain a high standard of oral cleanliness.

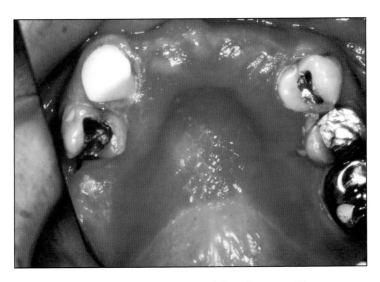

Figure 2.5 Denture stomatitis: red areas of the palate caused by contact with a partial upper denture. Patients rarely complain of soreness and may be completely unaware of the condition. It is mainly due to candidal infection and is associated with poor denture hygiene and wearing dentures at night

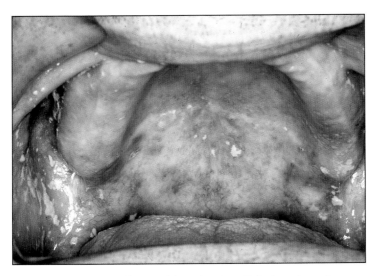

Figure 2.6 Candidal infection of the palate in a diabetic patient who wore a complete upper denture

Self-applied commercial soft linings and denture fixatives should generally not be used for long periods as they may mask underlying problems with the dentures. The linings can also act as a growth medium for micro-organisms.

A dry mouth (xerostomia) may be the cause of poor denture retention. A thin film of saliva provides much of the adhesion for an upper denture. A reline or remake may be indicated if the dentures are loose or ill fitting. The normal life expectancy of dentures is approximately five years, yet it is not uncommon to encounter dentures made decades previously (*Figure 2.7*).

Professionally fitted soft linings can improve comfort for some individuals who experience discomfort from the resorption of the bony ridges. Temporary soft linings have a limited life and often lose their elasticity and require replacement within two years.

Denture hygiene

Denture cleaners may be effective in removing staining, but long-term immersion is not indicated as these products have a bleaching effect. This will discolour the whole denture and many damage any soft linings. Special care is needed to clean soft linings in order to prevent premature hardening. The resilience of the soft lining may be affected by denture cleaning materials and the temperature of the water used.

Most proprietary denture cleaners, have some disadvantages (*Table 2.4*). Rinsing or soaking does not remove plaque efficiently and brushing is the only effective method.

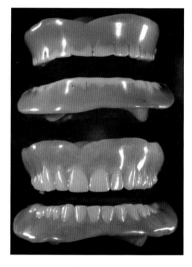

Figure 2.7 Old dentures and new dentures

Table 2.4 Denture cleaners

Denture cleaner	Method	Effect
Alkaline peroxides	Soaking	Do not readily remove stain
Hypochlorite	Soaking	May cause bleaching May corrode metal dentures Removes plaque well
Chlorhexidine	Soaking	May stain dentures Very effective against plaque
Dilute acids	Brush on	Effective for stain removal and heavy deposits May corrode metal dentures
Denture pastes	Brushing	Abrasive to denture plastic

Ultrasonic cleaning baths are useful for removing hard deposits of calculus.

Dentures should be left out of the mouth at night and stored in plain water or in a cleansing solution. A suitable cleansing solution is 1 part Milton 1% to 80 parts water for plastic dentures. For dentures with metal clasps, chlorhexidine 0.2% should be used[17].

Naming dentures

Marking dentures with the owner's name can help reunite the owner with their dentures if lost in a hospital or care setting. The most effective method is to incorporate the name at the stage of manufacture. It is possible to temporarily mark afterwards using a denture marking kit or covering an identifying mark with nail varnish, although this needs to be checked regularly and repeated. Anecdotal evidence about the communal cleaning of dentures in care settings is now fortunately rare due to changes in nursing practice but the loss of dentures for in-patients and residents is still a far too frequent occurrence.

2.13 Summary

For the self-caring adult, the basic principles and practice of oral care are elementary. The difficulties lie in that most people receive their knowledge from a wide variety of conflicting sources and follow habits and routines

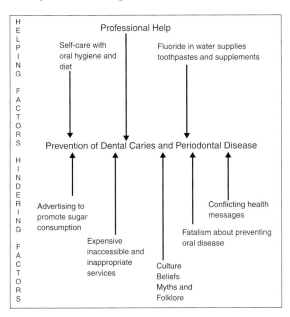

Figure 2.8 Helping and hindering factors in oral care

established over many years. These are difficult to modify in the light of new evidence based practices.

Many self-caring adults do not visit the dentist except when they perceive a need[16] and therefore do not receive up to date advice on oral care.

When other health threats upset self-care routines, personal and oral care may suffer. *Figure 2.8* summarises some of the common helping and hindering factors.

References

1. COMA. Department of Health. 1989 Dietary Sugars and Human Disease. Report of the Panel on Dietary Sugars of the Committee on Medical Aspects of Food Policy. Report 37. London. HMSO.

2. Diet, Nutrition and the Prevention of Chronic Diseases. WHO Technical Report Series 916. 2003. Report of a Joint WHO/FAO Expert Consultation. pp105-119. Geneva, WHO.

3. The Balance of Good Health. 2001. Food Standards Agency.

4. Screenivasan P, Gaffar A. Antiplaque biocides and bacterial resistance: a review. *J Clin Periodontol* 2002 **29**: 965-974.

5. Marthaler TM, O'Mullane DM, Vrbic V. The prevalence of dental caries in Europe 1990-1995. *Caries Res* 1996 **30**: 237-255.

6. Levine R, Stillman-Lowe C. The scientific basis of dental health education. 5th Edition. London: British Dental Journal Books, 2004.

7. Marinho VCC, Higgins JPT, Logan S *et al. Fluoride gels for preventing dental caries in children and adolescents (Cochrane Review)*. In: The Cochrane Library, Issue 2, 2002. Oxford.

8. Health Evidence Bulletins Wales. Oral Health. March 1998. Cardiff. Welsh Office.

9. Morris J, White D. The York review of water fluoridation-key points for the busy practitioner. *Dent Update*. 2000 **27**: 474-475.

10. The British Fluoridation Society. http://www.liv.ac.uk/bfs/

11. McCracken GI, Stacey F, Heasman L *et al.* A comparative study of two powered toothbrushes and one manual toothbrush in young adults. *J Clin Dent* 2001 **12**: 7-10.

12. Preston AJ. A review of dentifrices. *Dent Update* 1998 **25**: 247-253.

13. Ogden GR, Macluskey M. An overview of the prevention of oral cancer and diagnostic markers of malignant change: 1 Prevention. *Dent Update* 2000 **27**: 95-99.

14. Dhawan N, Bedi R. Transcultural oral health care: 6 The oral health of minority ethnic groups in the United Kingdom – a review. *Dent Update* 2001 **28**: 30-34.

15. Chestnutt IG, Binnie VI. Smoking cessation counselling- a role for the dental profession? *Br Dent J* 1995 **179**: 411-415.

16. Nuttall N, Steele JG, Nunn J *et al.* A Guide to the UK Adult Dental Health Survey 1998. London: British Dental Journal Books, 2001.

17. Sweeney MP, Bagg J. Making sense of the mouth. Partnerships in oral care. 1997. University of Glasgow Media Services www.gla.ac.uk/schools/dental

Chapter 3

Child oral health

3.1 Children as a special group

Traditionally, children have been identified as a special group at greater risk from dental and oral disease. This is due to society's perception of the dependent status of children who require special protection and provisions. In addition the onset of dental disease, particularly dental caries, during childhood in most industrialised societies results in a focus on children as a target group for prevention.

A number of socio-demographic changes underway will change these assumptions. The changing age structures in most industrialised countries will mean that the proportion of older people will increase as the birth rate declines[1]. It is likely that it is the older population who will pose the greatest treatment challenges to health care teams, including dental teams. However, despite these demographic population changes in the UK it is still of vital importance to prevent oral and dental disease during childhood, as it remains a major health problem for large sections of the child population. Establishing good oral health practises in childhood provides the foundations for oral health in adult life.

The initial high prevalence of dental diseases in children leads to a focus for dental services and allocation of resources to this group by many countries[2]. There is also a clear logic in establishing early practices of regular dental visits in childhood and the opportunity for primary prevention of dental disease. However, the reduction in the prevalence of dental caries seen in many industrialised societies will significantly reduce the overall treatment needs of children. But, the strong association of dental disease with aspects of deprivation and socio-economic factors is focussing the disease burden on different subgroups of children in the community. Although these groups have disproportionate levels of disease there is still a need to focus preventive and treatment services to all children across society[2].

The social, cultural and environmental aspects of dental disease may place children more at risk as dental caries begins with the widespread consumption throughout childhood of sugar and sugar containing products as pacifiers, bribes or rewards. Snacking between meals, which increases the risk of caries, is also part of the youth culture[3].

In developing countries, the caries rate is rising in those parts of the community with access to refined sugar products[4]. Although children are predominantly affected, as many countries have a much younger population, the whole community is at risk once the challenge to dental health has been introduced.

It should also be recognised that children should be considered in the context of their family and the family's susceptibility to dental and oral disease. This is affected by exposure to fluoride, dietary patterns in the family, use of dental services and the degree to which their families and communities value a preventive approach to oral health.

3.2 The need to establish prevention in childhood

Patterns of dental treatment needs and an individual's attitudes to oral health are partly shaped by childhood experiences. Routines established during childhood will form the basis of many of our adult behaviour patterns, based on the process of primary socialisation[5]. The stress and anxiety that affects many adults at dental visits are the result of traumatic dental visits in childhood. The trauma of extraction of primary teeth with a general anaesthetic is an often-cited example[6]. Early experience of dental caries and subsequent treatment will map out a person's treatment needs throughout adult life. Restorations will require replacement and inevitably become more complex. An individual's future treatment needs can be largely predicted from the state of their oral health when 12-14 years old[7].

3.3 The primary and secondary dentition

There are a number of anatomical differences between the primary and secondary dentition, but these do not intrinsically alter the susceptibility to dental caries. It is important for all health professionals to encourage a preventive approach at an early stage, during the primary dentition. This will combat a fatalism often encountered towards dental disease in the primary dentition as well as for the following sound reasons:

- To prevent pain
- To reduce the need for extractions and other interventions
- To prevent orthodontic complications in the secondary dentition *(Figure 3.1)*.

Early experiences of dental related pain and subsequent treatment, which may involve extraction of teeth will strongly contribute to producing a dentally anxious patient[6]. Early loss of primary teeth may also encourage the following secondary teeth to erupt in unfavourable positions, which can result in malocclusions and poor aesthetics. Crowded and malpositioned teeth will also be more difficult to clean effectively *(Figure 3.1)*.

Although the crowns of primary teeth are all fully developed at birth, the secondary permanent dentition starts to develop and calcify around this time *(Figure 3.2)*. Birth, or perinatal, trauma can result in malformations,

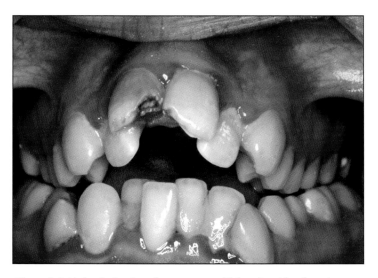

Figure 3.1 Malocclusion in a fourteen-year-old female with a learning difficulty. Early intervention to extract teeth would have reduced the degree of overcrowding, although orthodontic treatment would not have been appropriate due to poor compliance and co-operation. A fractured upper central tooth is decayed suggesting lack of dental treatment

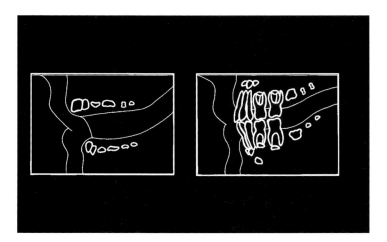

Figure 3.2 Primary teeth developing in the jaws of an unborn child (left) and secondary teeth developing above and below the primary teeth (right). Note, there is no primary tooth preceding the first permanent molar

sometimes seen as a distinctive line visible when the teeth erupt into the mouth from 6-7 years of age *(Figure 1.1)*. Untreated dental decay in primary teeth can result in malformations and damage to the permanent teeth, which are already developing underneath (*Figure 3.2*).

3.4 Formulating an oral preventive approach

Whichever method is used for planning and implementing a preventive approach, it is important to use a logical, planned approach which includes:

- Assessment
- Planning
- Implementation
- Evaluation.

This has parallels with the cyclical nursing process used in general nursing care.

3.5 Assessment

This usually starts with an interview with the parent or guardian. The first step in establishing sound preventive behaviour during childhood will take, as a starting point, the attitudes and beliefs of the parent or guardian. Their past experiences can sometimes result in a conflict between a wish for their children to avoid their own experiences, and a fatalism that their children will inevitably suffer dental disease. There are many variables that affect health-related behaviour; these can be sociological or part of the individual's psychological make-up. It is understandable that parents wish to avoid their child suffering pain and discomfort. But this, coupled with a negative attitude to the values of prevention and regular dental attendance, can encourage an avoidance of dental visits except for acute problems.

There is a tendency to predict the views of individuals by assuming that they hold the views of their socio-economic group. For example, it is commonly believed that people from some socio-economic groups are fatalistic about their health and see little value in prevention[8]. However, more detailed examination of groups show that more complex reasoning is taking place. An individual's decision making is influenced by the values of the family network, individual trust in health services and professionals, and past treatment[9]. Indeed, because of the complexity of predicting behaviour, it is better for the health professional to approach the practical situation with as few preconceptions as possible. It is valuable for the dental team to work closely with other members of the health care team in order for them to play their role in overcoming anxiety barriers by giving positive messages about the value of dental attendance.

3.6 Planning an holistic approach to prevention

Much of the health service in the UK is organised like a department store with separate sections for different organs, diseases and procedures. This reflects the views of the health professions about the body being compared to a machine with different components, rather than the everyday view of 'health' involving both body and mind.

This separation into specialities extends from treatment services into prevention and can become a barrier. Although it is reasonable to expect specialisation into different complex areas of medical interventions in order to ensure that the health professional providing care has a high level of skill, the reason for a division in labour becomes less clear in preventive approaches.

The actual core messages and approaches to the prevention of dental and oral disease are common to promoting good general health. This includes diet, smoking, hygiene and appropriate use of health services and, most importantly, promoting self-care and reliance.

Detecting the 'at-risk' individual

As described in Chapter 1, there is a general downward trend in dental disease in industrialised societies. However, there are still groups and individuals substantially at risk within particular communities. As these groups experience higher levels of disease compared to an improving background picture the 'health divide' becomes wider. As dental disease still has a very wide prevalence amongst children a 'whole population' approach to prevention is still required, with additional support for those at higher risk *(Figure 3.3)*.

Some of the factors that may place a child in a higher risk group include:

- Social group
- Ethnicity
- Geographical location
- Presence of existing dental disease
- Medical conditions
- Impairments.

Social group

There are inherent problems in predicting behaviour according to how

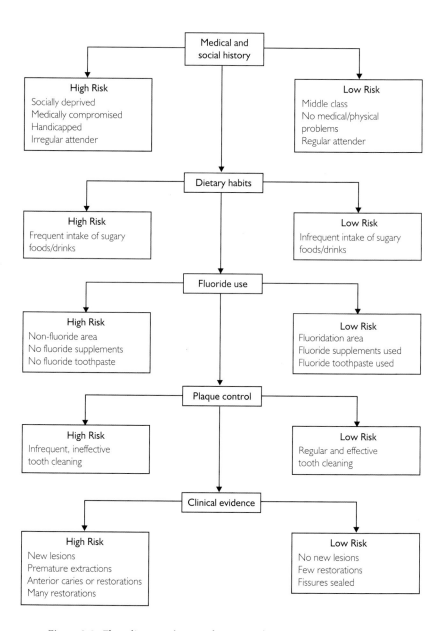

Figure 3.3 Flow diagram showing five types of data to be considered when assessing the caries risk of individual patients. (Reprinted from Positive Dental Prevention. The Prevention in childhood of dental disease in adult life Elderton RJ. p27. 1987 with permission from Elsevier)[10]

health professionals perceive a particular social group or class should behave. But there is no doubt that a greater understanding of an individual's social circumstances will help formulate a more suitable preventive approach. Using careful non-judgemental questioning, it is possible to ascertain the individual's current views and knowledge. This can act as a foundation on which to build a preventive approach. This will include an assessment of the value of oral health and the dental attendance pattern of the parent or guardian.

Ethnicity

There is wide reported variation in the dental health of children from differing ethnic groups[11]. Some of the factors which result in poorer dental health include social isolation, language barriers and some cultural practices associated with diet.

Geographical location

Although related to social class, the presence of other children, work commitments and poor public transport may create barriers that influence preventive regimes. The availability and types of local shopping can affect the provision of a healthy diet.

Presence of existing dental disease

A detailed dental examination will identify treatment needs. At this stage of planning, a preventive approach a parent's perception of perceived need, and even the views of an untrained eye may reveal the existence of untreated disease (*Figures 1.6 - 1.8*).

Medical conditions

The presence of other medical conditions may place a child more at risk from dental disease and dental treatment. Long term medications for children may not be available in sugar-free preparations and 'over the counter' medications may not be purchased as sugar-free alternatives. Chronically sick children may also be at risk as good dental health may be considered a low priority by parents or other health professionals[12].

Physical impairments

There are still widespread perceptions that children with a learning difficulty or a physical impairment are unable to receive routine dental care. Consequently, they may have delayed contacts with the preventive aspects of dental services. Although there is now a much more team approach to meeting all their needs, the dental team is often overlooked.

3.7 Implementing a practical preventive regime

After establishing the degree of risk, the key to success is to make a number of small changes over a period of time rather than attempting drastic alterations in routines that will not be maintained.

Dietary changes

Particularly for children with active dental caries, it is important to identify the number of sugar intakes. These include not only those in confectionery and added sugars but also 'hidden sugars' in fruit squashes and carbonated drinks. Often snack foods and drinks are high in sugar content. Since it is the frequency, or number of sugar intakes, which is crucial in the development of dental caries, a suitable strategy is the restriction of any sugar-containing products to mealtimes. A particularly high-risk time for young children is at night when they may be given a sugary drink in a feeder or a sugar dipped dummy.

Sugar is sometimes added to bottle feeds in the belief that the child will benefit from extra calories and the lay belief still persists that sugar in water is a relief for constipation. The distinctive pattern of decay on the front teeth caused by contact with sugar solutions, often referred to as 'bottle decay', can be seen in *Figure 1.6*. Due to conflicting information received from media advertising and unclear labelling, parents frequently fail to appreciate the hidden sugar content of foods and drinks. There are also long standing erroneous views that certain products are safer for children's teeth. An example being that white chocolate is less cariogenic than ordinary chocolate or that 'white' or clear lemonade is less harmful.

The other key strategy is the use of sugar substitutes in the diet. This refers not just to the use of artificial sweeteners, but also to the use of other rewards, such as toys, comics or books, instead of sweets or other sweet tasting foods. Artificial sweeteners are not recommended for children as they may cause gastric problems, except those specifically included in child products.

Sugar in drinks and confectionery form a significant part of dietary intake for all groups[13], none more so than young adults for whom consumption of such products is part of youth culture *(Figures 1.7 and 1.8)*. Decisions in youth, including patterns of sugar consumption, are very strongly affected by peer group pressure, which can override an individual's intentions not to consume sugar products on health grounds[14]. This desire to conform is used extensively in the advertising of sugar containing drinks and confectionery, which often portray models using these products.

Oral hygiene measures

Tooth brushing

There are two main reasons for tooth brushing:

- To remove plaque to prevent dental caries and periodontal disease
- To apply a daily dose of fluoride topically to teeth.

This is, of course, the rationale for tooth brushing from a medical perspective, while most individuals have the social goals of wanting clean teeth and fresh breath, as part of the grooming process[15].

The twice daily brushing of teeth varies considerably throughout countries, communities and with gender[16]. The variation can be partly explained by family socialisation patterns, which may be resistant to change. Other factors, such as family size and social class, can influence the frequency of tooth brushing among children and particularly adolescents[17]. As part of the assessment phase, the 'when and where' aspects of oral hygiene behaviour need to be established. Also, who has responsibility for supervising tooth brushing in the home and how it fits into the domestic routine.

Techniques for effective tooth brushing are the same for a child as for an adult (Chapter 2). The main difference is that children up to the age of seven years will require help, particularly in the posterior regions of the mouth, and the lingual and palatal surfaces. As part of the socialisation process it is important that young individuals have the opportunities to acquire and practice skills for themselves. Tooth brushing therefore becomes part teaching and part supervisory as the child becomes more proficient. *(Figures 3.4- 3.6).*

For tooth brushing to be effective in preventing dental disease, a small number of thorough brushings are better than frequent scant brushing. There is little to be gained by brushing after every meal, and for most children this would not be practical in many school and social environments.

Other oral hygiene measures

The use of dental floss can aid in removing plaque from between teeth. It does require a high level of manual dexterity and considerable practice before it can be used comfortably. Dental team members who are used to working intra-orally and with mirrors may underestimate the difficulty. Children do not really develop the required level of dexterity to use floss safely and efficiently until approximately 12-years-old. The use of floss should be taught on an individual basis by a member of the dental team and practised under supervision to avoid trauma to gum tissues.

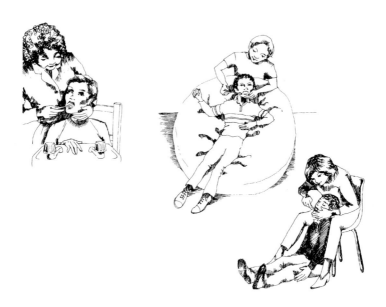

Figures 3.4 – 3.6 Positions for assisting a child

Toothbrushing is easier if approached from behind a child with head supported against the carer. It may be done from a standing, seated or kneeling position. The drawings show different methods which may be useful for children or disabled adults

Fluorides

The simplest, most effective way of administering fluoride is via the drinking water supply. This method has been shown to be safe and effective and has been in use for over fifty years in parts of the USA[18].

The next most important source of fluoride is via toothpaste. It is more difficult to control the amount of fluoride ingested by young children. A pea-sized amount should be used and the child encouraged to spit out to minimise the risk of 'mottling' or fluorosis of the enamel in the permanent teeth[19]. Topical fluorides can also be delivered as mouthwash or brush on gel for higher risk groups.

A high level of protection from dental caries can be given by systemic fluoride supplements. These can be given as drops for the youngest age groups and tablets for older children. It is important to view these supplements as a long-term measure to ensure that ongoing protection is given to enamel. For maximum effect, the daily supplement should be in contact with the teeth for as long as possible. Tablets should be sucked or chewed. If the supplement is taken at bedtime after brushing, the length of contact time with the teeth will be prolonged. The daily dosage for fluoride supplements for areas with less than 0.3ppm fluoride in the water supply is shown in *Table 2.3*[19].

All individuals should use fluoridated toothpaste on a daily basis. The decision to use extra supplements in low-fluoridated water areas depends on the following major risk factors:

- Individual and social susceptibility to dental caries based on a previous high level of caries in the primary dentition or a family history
- Risk of complications from the effects of chronic illness, dental disease or dental treatment
- Medical conditions where the individual is at reduced ability to combat infection
- Learning difficulties and other groups, who may experience additional barriers to receiving adequate oral and dental health care.

Dosages for fluoride supplements vary according to age and the fluoride content in the drinking water supply. Fluoride gels and varnishes can also be applied by a member of the dental team from two to four times a year depending on individual risk.

Regular dental visits

There is a wide variation in how often visits are made to the dentist when the reason is not for pain relief[20]. The factors involved in the decision to attend are a combination of whether there is a perceived need and the acceptability of the dental service. As a professional group, dentists have had encouraging success in mobilising considerable portions of society to attend regularly or to feel guilty if they do not[21].

There are a number of clear, evidence-based reasons, for regular attendance including;

- Monitoring the efficiency of plaque removal
- Early detection of caries to ensure more minimal interventions
- Early detection of orthodontic problems
- Screening for other disorders, including malignant and pre-malignant conditions.

As a baseline, a yearly examination should be the norm[22] but children should be seen more frequently during the stages of dental development.

Fissure sealants

Fissure sealants are resin coatings applied to the fissures of permanent molar teeth. As the fissures are inaccessible to tooth brushing the plaque which accumulates there renders them the most vulnerable sites for dental caries to develop. For children in high risk groups there are clear indications for the use of fissure sealants on permanent teeth[23]. They can be applied as soon as clinically possible after eruption or to sound teeth following an intervention for caries[23].

Oral trauma

Where there is a known risk of trauma to the permanent teeth, for example in contact sports, a mouth guard should be worn. To ensure an accurate fit these should be constructed by the dental team and may need changing as the jaw develops. However, oral trauma can also occur during normal play and social activities. Agencies involved in the care of children including schools, youth centres and sports clubs should have information and provide training in dental first aid and how to deal with damaged and avulsed teeth. Basic first aid advice for an avulsed tooth should include:

- Find the tooth and always hold it by the crown
- If the tooth is clean, replant it
- If the tooth is dirty, rinse in milk or cold water before replanting
- Secure the tooth in place, asking the child to bite on a handkerchief
- Visit a dentist as soon as possible.

If the tooth cannot be replanted immediately:

- Store in plain milk
- Alternatively, the tooth can be stored in the patient's mouth if appropriate
- Do not allow the tooth to dry out nor store it in any other medium, including disinfectants.

All health professionals should be aware of non-accidental injury presenting as oral trauma. All health communities have policies and procedures for child protection and any suspicion of abuse should be discussed with colleagues and documented. Advice should be sought from child health protection professionals or duty social workers. Where there is clear disclosure of abuse or strong suspicions, an immediate referral to social services is indicated.

3.8 Evaluating a preventive regime

A number of health outcome criteria can be used to evaluate the preventive approach but because dental disease can progress relatively slowly it can take several years to see evidence of results. As most preventive methods are linked to behaviour change, it is possible to monitor effectiveness via a series of observed or reported changes. These could be changes in dietary practices, improvements in oral hygiene or increased use of dental services.

Unfortunately, the dental profession has often used fear-arousal as a motivating factor, and this has led to a tendency for people to be less open in their accounts of dental health behaviour.

Several indicators of good gingival health can be used to evaluate the effectiveness of oral hygiene measures. These include the absence of bleeding when brushing, as well as the colour and appearance of the gingival tissues.

3.9 Summary

There are clear indications for establishing a preventive regime during childhood. The plan should include four broad phases:

- Assessment
- Planning
- Implementation
- Evaluation.

References

1. Census 2001. Ageing population. National Statistics Online. http://www.statistics.gov.uk/ 2003.

2. Chen M, Andersen RM, Barmes DE et al. Comparing Oral Health Care Systems. A Second International Collaborative Study. p52. Geneva: World Health Organisation, 1997.

3. Changing food culture. promoting health. J Health Promotion Northern Ireland June 2003.

4. Lo ECM, Holmgren CJ, Hu De-yu et al. Dental caries status and treatment needs of 12–13-year-old children in Sichuan Province, Southwestern China. Community Dent Health 1999 16: 114-116.

5. Freeman R. The psychology of dental patient care. p37-45. London: British Dental Association, 2000.

6. Milsgrom P, Weinstein P. Dental fears in general practice: new guidelines for assessment and treatment. Int Dent J 43: 288-293.

7. Murray JJ. The potential for prevention in children. In Elderton RJ(Ed). Positive dental prevention. The prevention in childhood of dental disease in adult life. p4.Oxford: Heineman, 1987.

8. Davis, P Introduction to the sociology of dentistry. p31. Otago: Otago Press, 1980.

9. Bennett P, Murphy S. Psychology and health promotion. p23. Open University Press, 1997.

10. Elderton RJ. Positive Dental Prevention. The prevention in childhood of dental disease in adult life. p27. Oxford, Heinmann, 1987.

11. Dhawan N, Bedi R. Transcultural oral health care: 6 The oral health of minority ethnic groups in the United Kingdom – a review. *Dent Update* 2001 **28**: 30-34.

12. Nunn J. Disability and oral care. Ed. Nunn J. p11. London: FDI World Dental Press Ltd., 2000.

13. COMA. Department of Health. 1989 Dietary Sugars and Human Disease. Report of the Panel on Dietary Sugars of the Committee on Medical Aspects of Food Policy. Report 37. London. HMSO.

14. Traeen B, Rise J. Dental health behaviours in a Norwegian population. *Community Dent Health* 1990 **7**: 59-68.

15. Hodge HC, Holloway PJ, Bell CR. Factors associated with tooth brushing behaviour in adolescents. *Br Dent J* 1982 **152**: 49-51.

16. Chen M, Andersen RM, Barmes D *et al.* Comparing oral health care systems. A second international collaborative study. p75 Geneva: World Health Organisation, 1997.

17. MacGregor IDM. Tooth brushing frequency in relation to family size and bedtimes in English schoolchildren. *Community Dent Oral Epidemiol* 1987 **15**:181-183.

18. Morris J, White D. The York review of water fluoridation-key points for the busy practitioner. *Dent Update* 2000 **27**: 474-475.

19. Levine R, Stillman-Lowe C. The scientific basis of dental health education. 5th Ed. p33. London: British Dental Association, 2004.

20. Nuttall N, Steele JG, Nunn J *et al.* Guide to the UK Adult Dental Health Survey 1998. p35. London: British Dental Association, 2001.

21. Davis, P Introduction to the sociology of dentistry. p91. Otago: Otago Press, 1980.

22. National Clinical Guidelines and Policy Documents 1999. p18. Faculty of Dental Surgery of the Royal College of Surgeons of England Clinical Effectiveness Committee. Dental Practice Board.

23. National Clinical Guidelines and Policy Documents 1999. p6. Faculty of Dental Surgery of the Royal College of Surgeons of England Clinical Effectiveness Committee. Dental Practice Board.

Chapter 4

Oral health care for older people

4

4.1 Introduction

General health care is important for all ages. Good oral hygiene is a vital aspect of health care and a comfortable healthy mouth is as important for older people as for any other section of the population. For those experiencing illness, impairment or disability, maintaining a healthy mouth may make a significant contribution to the process of rehabilitation and recovery.

The impact of oral conditions on individuals' quality of life can be profound[1,2]. Older people experience the same oral and dental problems as the general population but oral problems have a significant effect on well-being and life satisfaction in older people with chronic physical and mental conditions which may add an additional burden[3]. However, good oral health can contribute holistically towards improvements in general health, social acceptability, self-esteem and quality of life[1,4].

Care of the mouth is an essential part of personal daily care. Primary health care professionals are in a position to encourage older people to take good care of their mouths, to promote and to maintain oral health. It is their role to motivate, support, assist or provide oral care if the individual is functionally dependent. They are therefore in a prime position to identify oral problems which may go unnoticed unless the individual is seeing a dentist regularly.

The mouth and associated structures play an important physiological role in mastication and nutrition. However the social importance of the mouth in both speech and appearance is often a neglected aspect of care for older people. The ability to communicate and the dignity and self-esteem given by self-confidence in one's appearance have obvious psychological benefits. Aside from systemic benefits, a nourishing and well-balanced diet contributes to general health and well-being.

With the onset of illness, deterioration in the ability to manage personal care can lead to a cycle of problems associated with neglect, which may cause a change in diet leading to poor nutritional intake and further physical deterioration. A mouth ulcer, sharp tooth or loose dentures may contribute to, or even precipitate, a change in diet. These problems can usually be treated quite easily if identified at an early stage.

In order to achieve the objective of a comfortable healthy mouth it is helpful to have some understanding of the oral and dental problems of older people and the barriers, both real and perceived that they may experience in obtaining dental care and maintaining oral health.

4.2 Demography, impairment and disability

It is a well known fact that the UK population is ageing. The Government's projections suggest that by 2020, the population will reach 63.9 million and peak in 2040 at around 66 million[5]. The proportion of older people is expected to rise. Although the 'baby boomers' of the 1940s and 1960s are an important factor, the main reasons are longer life expectancy and a fall in mortality in older age groups[6]. Over the next ten years, the increase in numbers of old and very old people in society will exceed that for the population as a whole. By 2020, more than 12 million people of pensionable age will be living in the UK, with twice as many females as males over the age of 85. The UK population of older people is not a homogenous group. It will also be more ethnically and culturally diverse as second and third generations of immigrants reach older age.

In discussing the needs of older people and their use of services, the increase in impairment and disability with age must be considered. The 1988 OPCS survey, the first of its kind in the UK to look at this from a functional rather than a medical perspective, estimated that 6.2 million of the adult population of Great Britain, of which 4.2 million were aged 60 or more, had a level of 'disability' above that laid down by criteria for the survey[7]. The overall rate of 'disability' increased with age, accelerating after the age of 50 years. 'Disability' rose very steeply over the age of 70, with almost 70% of 'disabled' adults aged over 60, and almost 50% aged 70 or over. The most severely 'disabled' lived in residential or institutional care. Mobility was the most frequently reported functional problem with hearing impairment and the inability to manage personal care affecting more than a third of 'disabled' people. In the 60–74 age group, approximately 20% were estimated to have impaired mobility, rising to 46% in those aged over 75.

More recent reports confirm that long-term illness limits the lifestyle of over a third of the population aged 65 to 74, and almost half the population over 75, particularly:

- Loss of mobility increases with age
- The greatest decline in mobility is in people aged 75 and over
- Sensory impairments become more common as people age
- Around 80% of people over 60 have a visual impairment
- 75% of people over 60 have a hearing impairment
- 22% have both visual and hearing impairment[8,9].

The numbers with cognitive impairment will increase because the chances of developing dementia rise sharply with age. The Alzheimer's Society estimates that there are currently 700,000 people in the UK with dementia[10]. The majority are aged 65 years or older. However progress in the understanding of conditions such Alzheimer's disease may lead to developments in its prevention and treatment so predictions must be viewed with caution.

The National Service Framework for Older People distinguishes between people who are functionally independent and those who are functionally dependent or frail regardless of age[11]. This classification is used in 2020 Vision which looks at the current and future oral health needs of older people in the UK and makes wide reaching recommendations for oral health care[12]. But it is the frail or functionally dependent population of older people who are the primary concern of this chapter.

Effective mouth care requires perceptuo-motor skill and manual dexterity. Older people who are active and independent should have little difficulty maintaining oral health. However functional impairment will pose limitations on the management of personal oral hygiene and is likely to severely restrict access to dental care and information on services. The Government's report, *Access to NHS Dentistry* confirms the fact that older people and people with dementia experience particular problems accessing NHS dental care[13]. Older people in residential care do not receive uniformly high standards of oral health care[14] and this is confirmed by a number of studies[14-18]. Guidelines to address these issues provide a framework for developing standards to improve oral health in residential care settings[4].

Older people tend to have a much greater need for health and social care services. Most of those who are frail or functionally dependent are living at home and therefore less easily identifiable except through contact with statutory and voluntary agencies. The proportion living in residential or continuing care facilities are more easily identified. The introduction of annual, general medical practitioner surveillance for the over 75s provided an opportunity to identify and screen for oral problems. Implementation of the 'Single Assessment Process'[11] and the 'Unified Assessment'[19] provide an opportunity to include a basic oral health risk assessment into a comprehensive and holistic assessment process. A simple questionnaire has successfully alerted health care professionals to oral and dental problems[20,21]. Examples can be found in Chapter 6. Assessment for oral health care and individual care plans are now a requirement across all health and social care settings in Wales[22], for example. If implemented, the recommendations for a free oral health assessment for people over 60 with referral for a strategic long-term oral health care plan and basic local standards for oral health in residential care[12] will have a very positive impact on the oral health of frail and functionally dependent older people.

4.3 Oral effects of ageing

Tooth loss is not an inevitable consequence of ageing, although there are changes in oral tissues and surrounding structures associated with the ageing process. The degree of change depends on a variety of individual factors:

- Genetic influences
- Lifestyle
- Habits
- Experience of disease
- Nutrition.

Teeth

Tooth structure undergoes changes with age. Attrition, loss of tooth substance through wear, is related to diet, habits such as bruxism (grinding teeth), and to the extra load that is placed upon the remaining teeth when some teeth have been lost (*Figure 4.1*). Attrition of the biting surfaces may lead to loss of facial height, although this is sometimes compensated for by an extra deposit of cement around the roots (hypercementosis).

Enamel may also be lost due to erosion (*Figure 2.3*) or abrasion as a result of excessive or incorrect brushing techniques (*Figure 2.4*). Abrasion is most

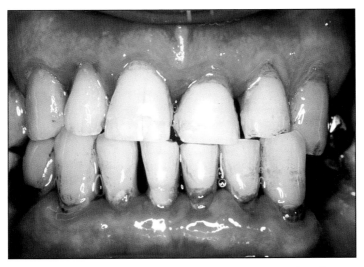

Figure 4.1 An 88-year-old self-caring male retaining most teeth with some recession of the gingivae and toothbrush abrasion at the gingival margins. The biting surfaces show attrition and there is some evidence of gingivitis. However, this is a relatively healthy mouth. The subject wears a skeleton design, cobalt chrome (metal) denture to restore occlusal contact

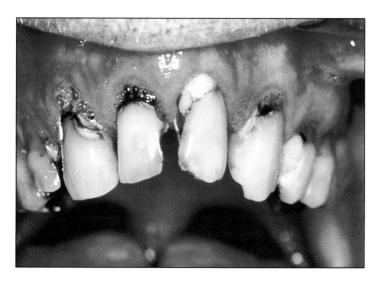

Figure 4.2 An elderly male whose oral and dental problems were identified as a result of admission to hospital following a cerebrovascular accident. There are signs of gingival recession, cervical (root) caries and deficient fillings

pronounced at the cervical surface (neck) of the tooth where the gum may have receded. Enamel also appears to darken with age due to the formation of additional layers of dentine within the tooth structure. The overall effect is that teeth become less sensitive to external stimuli.

Decay occurs more frequently in exposed root surfaces (root caries) (*Figure 4.2*). It is thought to be due to gingival recession (receding gums) exposing dentine which covers the root surface. Dentine is less resistant to caries than enamel, and together with poor oral hygiene and a soft diet create ideal conditions for root caries, the characteristic pattern of dental caries in older people.

Changes in structure with age make teeth more brittle. This increases the risk of fracture, particularly during extraction. Deposits of cementum around the roots may create complications for extractions and these are important considerations in planning dental treatment.

Bone

Age changes in bone affect the maxilla, mandible and other facial bones. Increased porosity and bone resorption follow tooth loss which leads to a greater potential for fracture. The cortical (surface) bone becomes thinner and in many older people, loss of bony ridges to support and stabilise a denture leads to difficulty in wearing dentures, particularly in the lower jaw.

Bone previously affected by periodontal disease is resorbed more quickly. Loss of function and wearing dentures that are entirely supported by soft tissue rather than by teeth can also contribute to increased bone loss. The changes described predispose to fracture and delayed healing, which have implications for dental treatment, leading to greater difficulty in construction of stable dentures.

Oral tissues

Mucous membranes generally atrophy with age. The rate at which this occurs in the mouth depends on diet, habits, denture wear and oral hygiene. The epithelium covering the cheeks and lips tends to become more keratinised, while the palate becomes less keratinised. Thinner oral mucosa is more easily damaged and penetrated by food substances and medication which may give rise to an itching or burning sensation.

Saliva and salivary glands

There is a considerable body of evidence to demonstrate the impact of salivary flow on oral health; with a lower flow rate the composition of saliva appears to have fewer protective properties. Changes in structure of the salivary glands are recorded and medication and salivary gland disease may reduce salivary flow, leading to dry mouth (xerostomia). Side-effects of medication are covered in Chapter 8. Age and medication are significant risk factors for xerostomia but medication is a better predictor of risk status than age[23]. The onset of xerostomia is associated with an increase in other oral symptoms, and problems with eating, communication and social interaction[24]. Thinner oral mucosa and a reduction in saliva can lead to serious problems that have an impact on an individual's quality of life.

Summary

Oral changes that occur as part of the ageing process or as a result of oral disease may give rise to considerable oral pain or discomfort. The immediate effect may cause a change in dietary habits that affects nutritional status with potentially negative consequences for general health. Age-changes associated with the mouth and oral tissues also have consequences for the planning and delivery of dental care.

4.4 Oral status

In 1968, 63% of the adult UK population were dentate, whereas the 1998 Adult Dental Health Survey reported that 87% of all adults had some natural teeth[25]. If the trend continues it is predicted that by 2028, the percentage with some natural teeth will rise to 96%. A small but varied group of people will continue to become edentulous (no natural teeth).

assumed and expected. One of the purposes of this book is to equip care providers with the necessary knowledge to deliver adequate oral health care for dependent people.

4.6 Barriers to oral health care

Decreased perception of oral problems (subjective need) and low awareness of the benefits of oral health compared with the dental profession's assessment of need (normative need) pose barriers to oral health. Past dental experiences and dental attendance patterns, habits, lack of knowledge, inaccurate beliefs, and professional attitudes, as well as much more practical factors such as cost, transport, illness, impaired mobility and dependence for personal care are contributory factors. By contrast, the 'young-old' who are better informed regarding oral health care, are more likely to have benefited from advanced techniques and express higher levels of subjective need based on positive dental experiences.

The belief that tooth loss is an inevitable consequence of ageing is probably due to restricted dental services in their youth and the practice of extractions with provision of dentures as the norm. A commonly held belief in dentures that will last a life-time as the ultimate solution to years of dental pain should gradually diminish (*Figure 2.7*). The practice of fathers paying for extractions and dentures as a dowry for their daughter is more than anecdotal among general dental practitioners in South Wales; but fortunately this practice now seems to be dying out.

Negative comments such as 'wasting the dentist's time' or not wishing to 'bother the dentist' are not anecdotal. It may be that negative attitudes to dental care are associated with negative stereotypes of ageing and repeated experience of ageism from professionals. Older people are now more concerned with preserving their teeth and the long-term value of oral healthcare[25]. Greater awareness of the benefits of oral health in 'middle-aged' groups who are more likely to retain teeth, who are themselves approaching retirement, and who are more likely to make demands for services, may result in a reduction in negative beliefs about oral health and benefits of dental care.

There is no simple classification that will cover the complexity of barriers to oral health. However they can be broadly grouped as patient, carer or professional related.

Table 4.2 Barriers to oral health[4,26,32]

Patient related barriers

Cost of dental treatment, particularly for socio-economic groups on low incomes

Real and perceived cost of treatment

Fear and apprehension about dental treatment

Decreased perception of oral health problems in geriatric populations

Inability to articulate need

Dependence on carers to identify need

Access to dental services due to physical impairment, transport difficulties or lack of an escort

Lack of knowledge of dental services and the availability of domiciliary care

Carer related barriers

Deficiencies in knowledge of basic oral hygiene among health professionals and carers

Family members and care staff placing dental care as a low priority

Limitations of workloads on long term care staff

Chronic inadequate oral hygiene practices

Lack of information on accessing dental care and domiciliary dental care

Dental related barriers

Older patients less likely to receive restorative treatment than younger patients

Lower socio-economic groups less likely to receive advanced dental care

Attitudes of dentist towards older people

Negative stereotypes of older people

Previous dental attendance patterns that influence treatment options

Poor confidence in treating older patients

Physical access and services within dental premises

Limitations of domiciliary dental care due to cost of equipment

Inadequate financial remuneration for domiciliary care

Dental attendance

Approximately 66% of the population aged 55 and over attend for regular dental care[25], and 58% of males and 78% of females in the 65-74 age group attend regularly compared with 64% and 57% respectively in the over 75s.

However, access to oral healthcare due to restricted mobility and other health problems will continue to be an issue for the frail or functionally dependent[12]. Since October 1999, dental service providers have had to take reasonable steps to change policies, practises and procedures that make it impossible or unreasonably difficult for a disabled person to use the service by providing reasonable alternatives[33]. Part III of the Disability Discrimination Act, which came into force in October 2004, requires dental service providers to make reasonable adjustments by removing or altering physical barriers within premises that make it impossible or unreasonably difficult for a disabled person to access dental care.

Cultural barriers

Ethnic minority communities are less likely to visit a dentist regularly except when in pain[34]. Lack of dental experience in older people who are immigrants from countries with less developed health care systems may be a contributory factor. However, risk behaviours such as smoking, or chewing tobacco, betel quid or pan are more common among certain ethnic groups[35]. Oral pathology is therefore likely to be diagnosed at a more advanced stage if dental attendance is prompted by the need for pain relief. Barriers relate to language, communication and lack of knowledge of cultural beliefs and practises. Although ethnic groups form a culturally diverse and small proportion of the elderly population in the UK, there is a danger of overlooking their differing health needs and problems.

Summary

The barriers described give some insight into why older people in the UK tend to visit the dentist less frequently with increasing age; similar barriers are identified throughout North America and Europe. With regular advice and support from professionals and carers, most older people would benefit from professional oral health care. Sensitivity to the needs of older people and the barriers quoted must be considered in attempting to change patterns of oral health behaviour and ensure appropriate access to dental services.

4.7 Routine check-ups

Regular oral examination is effective in screening for oral disease and oral cancers that have greater prevalence with advancing age (*Figure 1.11-1.13*). Prognosis is much improved with early diagnosis. Long-standing irritation from dentures (*Figure 4.3*) or a sharp tooth may increase the risk. Ulcers persisting for more than two weeks should be examined by a dentist. Potential premalignant conditions can be treated and monitored. This may involve advice on denture use and hygiene, adjusting dentures to prevent irritation, or smoothing a sharp-edged tooth. Counselling on risk

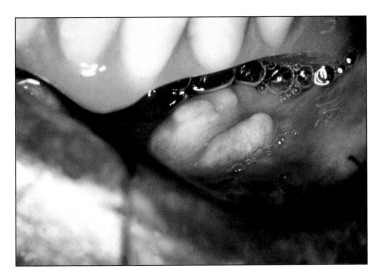

Figure 4.3 Denture granuloma caused by ill-fitting dentures

behaviour may be necessary, and information on risk behaviour should be more freely available. Screening for oral cancer is perhaps the most important reason for encouraging annual check-ups in this age group.

An annual check-up is recommended for all adults; this applies to individuals with no natural teeth or dentures. Hard and soft tissues can be examined and dentures checked to ensure they fit well and are not causing soft tissue damage. At the same time, the mouth is screened for oral and/or systemic diseases which exhibit oral signs or symptoms.

4.8 Oral care

Given the high oral health needs in frail or functionally dependent older people, it is very likely that such needs could be identified in older people in contact with health or social care services. A single question as to current registration with a dentist, or whether they have seen a dentist in the last year, may be all that is needed to identify those in need (Chapter 6). There will be local variation in the organisation of dental services (Chapter 5) and procedures for referral. The Primary Care Trust, Local Health Board or Community Dental Service should be contacted for advice on dental services in each locality.

The principles and practice of oral care for a self-caring individual apply; care of the teeth, mouth and dentures are described in detail in Chapter 2. Dietary reduction of refined sugars and effective plaque control are essential as any reduction in salivary flow increases the risk of dental caries, periodontal disease and oral infections. A reduction in salivary flow may be exacerbated by the xerostomic side-effects of medication[23].

When self-care deteriorates, practical advice and assistance will be required[22]. Encouragement may be all that is necessary as a prompt for self-care. However dependent older people who cannot carry out effective oral hygiene techniques will be reliant on a carer, whether professional or otherwise for this personal need.

Practical aspects of oral care

Oral tissues may be thin, inelastic, and more susceptible to damage with increasing age, so care must be taken in providing oral care. A small, soft, multi-tufted nylon tooth brush used gently but systematically is advisable. When providing oral care for the dependent person, the individual should be seated, and the head supported gently against the body for all techniques, whether tooth brushing, towelling or swabbing. Oral care for people who are highly dependent or dysphagic is described in Chapter 18[36]. If tooth brushing is difficult, teeth can be towelled with gauze wrapped around a gloved finger and soaked in chlorhexidine gluconate mouthwash or gel. This will help to control plaque and sweep away food debris from teeth and soft tissues but it is no substitute for tooth brushing.

Chemical plaque control

The bacterial content of plaque can be effectively reduced by chlorhexidine gluconate (Chapter 9). This may be used as an adjunct to tooth brushing and to reduce plaque on dentures. However it should not be used concurrently with toothpaste. Chorhexidine is very beneficial for plaque control for individuals who are at greater risk of oral or dental disease due to medical or behavioural problems, or when tooth brushing is difficult due to poor cooperation.

Mouth care

Dentures are worn by most people who have lost their natural teeth. Dentures facilitate mastication and help maintain a normal diet, thereby aiding nutrition, digestion and elimination. The choice of wearing dentures is of course up to the individual. However, many people seem to manage to eat satisfactorily with only one denture or even no dentures. The success of any treatment to construct new dentures depends largely on the individual's ability to cooperate in treatment and their motivation to wear dentures. If the individual is able to eat adequately and does not want dentures, then his or her decision should be respected, although counselling and advice may sometimes help them to see the benefits. The construction of an upper 'social' denture may provide a solution to the family's concerns.

Whether dentures are or are not worn, the mouth needs to be cleansed. The mouth should be rinsed after meals to remove food debris. The soft tissues and palate should be brushed with a small soft toothbrush. If these techniques cannot be tolerated, then all surfaces of the mouth should be wiped with gauze using a sweeping action to remove all food debris and this should be possible even if there is limited cooperation for oral care. Food tends to pouch in the sulci (area between cheek and gums), so particular attention should be paid to these areas.

Care of dentures

This is also covered comprehensively in Chapter 2. If dentures are worn at night, both mouth and dentures must be scrupulously clean. The importance of removing dentures at night cannot be over stressed. Night denture wearers are prone to develop candidal infections of soft tissues (*Figure 2.6*) or denture stomatitis (*Figure 2.5*), sometimes called 'denture sore mouth' (see also Chapter 15). This is exacerbated by plaque and poor denture hygiene. It can sometimes be difficult to break a long-standing habit of wearing dentures at night.

Dentures become coated with food and plaque. Plaque is not easily visible until quite a thick deposit has formed over a number of days. Hard deposits of calculus (tartar) may form in plaque deposits. This makes the surface rough and unhygienic, possibly causing irritation. The wearer may be unaware of the slowly accumulating deposit. The points to remember about denture care are:

- Remove dentures after meals
- Brush with a tooth or denture brush
- Use ordinary un-perfumed household soap
- Clean over a basin of cold water (to avoid accidental fracture if dropped)
- Rinse well before replacing in the mouth.

Soaking alone does not remove plaque, which is only effectively removed by brushing. Other points to remember in regularly handling dentures are:

- Check for rough or sharp areas
- Check for hard deposits
- Check whether dentures are marked with the owner's name for identification
- Refer to a dentist for the removal of stains or hard deposits of calculus.

Dentures that are unhygienic, old or worn may damage the delicate oral tissues and give rise to soreness, ulceration and infection. Chronic denture inflammation may predispose to potentially malignant oral pathology (*Figures 1.13 and 4.3*). If an area of soreness or ulceration persists, referral for a dental examination is essential.

A cycle of denture related problems is associated with illness in the older population. Initially the individual may have a reduced ability to cope with dentures or a reduced tolerance to wearing them. Oral or denture hygiene may be neglected and increasingly dentures are not worn, leading to dietary changes, poor nutritional intake and further physical deterioration. A dental opinion should be requested.

Dentures that have been worn successfully for many years are usually very acceptable to the wearer, rather like a comfortable pair of old slippers, even though the artificial teeth may be worn and alveolar ridges resorbed so that the dentures no longer fit. Over time, the wearer acclimatises to the changes unaware that their dentures no longer fit. Problems such as this tend to be identified following a stroke when facial paralysis leads to loss of neuromuscular control.

Minor adjustments to improve the fit with temporary or permanent soft lining are relatively simple and effective procedures to improve denture stability and retention. If changes are well tolerated, the existing dentures can be copied, eliminating unsatisfactory features but retaining the general shape and position of the teeth. It is often the best method of providing replacement or new dentures for people who have acclimatised to their old dentures. Denture construction is one of the most difficult technical areas of dentistry; it requires a reasonable level of comprehension and cooperation from the patient, whose physical or mental state may interfere with treatment or make it impossible to construct dentures. Dentures can however be modified to reduce the effect of facial paralysis by enlarging the denture on the affected side, helping to restore facial contour and reduce drooling.

Identification of dentures

Perhaps one of the biggest problems encountered by the dental profession is the request for replacement of lost dentures. New dentures should be marked with the wearer's name during construction. This is not universally practised but should be requested when new dentures are being constructed. Admission to hospital or residential accommodation is often accompanied by confusion and disorientation, and dentures may be lost, misplaced or even confused with those of another resident. Fortunately the misguided practice of collecting dentures and cleaning them together is now rare in continuing care, as large dormitory wards are being replaced by smaller units, but is a practice experienced by the authors. It can be difficult if not impossible to identify the correct owner of dentures.

Marking dentures with the owner's name is good practice and should be established as a standard procedure on admission to any form of communal establishment[4]. It does not prevent the loss of dentures but if found, they can be returned to the owner. Marking dentures discreetly near the posterior margins is a simple and cheap technique that takes a few minutes. It is preferably done with the resident's consent, pointing out the benefits of the technique. A denture marking kit, which can also be used to mark spectacles, is described in Chapter 9.

Tooth brushing aids

Aids to assist with gripping a tooth or denture brush, for people with reduced manual dexterity, or a change in use of the dominant hand are described in detail in Chapter 9. Simple adaptations include increasing the width of the handle, lengthening or bending the handle or by the attachment of aids such as a palm strap. The dental team and occupational therapist should have this advice available.

4.9 Summary

Oral and dental conditions 'handicap' older people[1]. Improving the oral and dental health of the older population is a major objective of the dental profession[12]. A high level of need has been identified in local and national surveys. Dental services that are tailored to the needs and wants of the individual must address the barriers described. Identifying frail and dependent individuals can only be achieved by an outreach approach in liaison with health, social care and voluntary agencies who provide care and support for older people[4]. As with children, older people are also vulnerable to abuse; health professionals should be aware of non-accidental injury to facial or oral tissues, and contact the appropriate authority with their concerns.

By providing information on the oral health needs of older people, the availability of appropriate dental services and the principles and practice of good oral care, it is anticipated that primary health care professionals will be better equipped to identify problems, provide appropriate oral care and access dental services.

References

1. Locker D. The burden of oral disorders in populations of older adults. *Community Dent Health* 1992 **9**: 109-124.

2. McGrath C, Bedi R. A study of the impact of oral health on the quality of life of older people in the UK - findings from a national survey. *Gerodontology* 1998 **15**: 93-98.

3. Locker D *et al.* Oral health-related quality of life of a population of medically compromised elderly people. *Community Dent Health* 2002 **19**: 90-97.

4. Fiske J, Griffiths J, Jamieson R *et al.* Guidelines for oral health care for long-stay patients and residents. *Gerodontology* 2000 **17**: 55-64.

5. Government Actuary's Department. Population Projections 2000-2070. London: GAD, 2002.

6. Tinker A. Ageing in the United Kingdom – what does this mean for dentistry? *Br Dent J* 2003 **194**: 369-372.

7. Martin, J., Meltzer, H, Elliott, D. The prevalence of disability among adults: Report I. 1998. London, OPCS Social Survey Division, HMSO.

8. Office for National Statistics. Social Trends 29. Edited by Matheson J and Pullinger J. The Stationary Office: London, 1999.

9. Living in Britain (1994). Making Sense (Appendix A) Redhouse Lane Publishing.

10. Alzheimer's Society. Facts about dementia. 2003. www.alzheimers.org.uk

11. Department of Health. National Service Framework for Older People. London: DoH, 2001.

12. BDA Monograph: Oral Healthcare for Older People: 2020 Vision. British Dental Association, 2003.

13. House of Commons, Health Committee. Access to NHS Dentistry: First Report. London: The Stationary Office, 2001.

14. Department of Health. NHS Dentistry: Options for Change. London: DoH, 2002.

15. Frenkel H, Harvey I, Newcombe RG. Oral health among nursing home residents in Avon. *Gerodontology* 2000 **17**: 33-38.

16. Simons D, Kidd EAM, Beighton D. Oral health of elderly residents in residential homes. *Lancet* 1999 **353**: 1761.

17. Longhurst R. An evaluation of the oral care given to patients when staying in hospital. *Primary Dent Care* 1999 **6**: 112-115.

18. McNally L, Gosney MA, Doherty U *et al.* The orodental status of a group of elderly in-patients: a preliminary assessment. *Gerodontology* 1999 **16**: 81-84.

19. Wales Assembly Government. Health and Social Care for Adults: Creating a unified and fair system for assessing and managing care. 2002.

20. Hoad-Reddick G. Assessment of elderly people on entry to residential homes and continuing care arrangements. *J Dent* 1992 **20**: 199-201.

21. Griffiths J. Guidelines for oral health care for people with a physical disability. *J Disabil Oral Health.* 2002 **3**: 51-58.

22. Welsh Assembly Government. Fundamentals of Care: Guidance for Health and Social Care Staff. 2003.

23. Field EA, Fear S, Higham SM *et al.* Age and medication are significant risk factors for xerostomia in an English population attending general dental practice. *Gerodontology* 2001 **18**: 21-24.

24. Locker D. Xerostomia in older adults: a longitudinal study. *Gerodontology* 1995 **12**: 18-25.

25. Kelly M, Steele J, Nuttall N *et al.* Adult Dental Health Survey: Oral Health in the UK in 1998. London, TSO, 2000.

26. Walls AW, Steele JG. Geriatric oral health issues in the United Kingdom. *Int Dent J* 2001 **51**: 183-187.

27. Todd J, Lader D. Adult Dental Health in the United Kingdom in 1988. London: HMSO, 1991.

28. Nunn J, Morris J, Pine C *et al.* The condition of teeth in the UK in 1998 and implications for the future. *Br Dent J* 2000 **189**: 639-643.

29. Steele JG, Walls, AW, Ayatollahi SM *et al.* Major clinical findings from a dental survey of elderly people in three different English communities. *Br Dent J* 1996 **180**: 17-23.

30. Samaranayake LP, Wilkieson CA, Lamey P *et al.* Oral disease in the elderly in long-term hospital care. *Oral Dis* 1995 **1**: 147-151.

31. Dormenval V, Budtz-Jorgensen E, Mojon P, *et al.* Nutrition, general health status and oral health status in hospitalised elders. *Gerodontology* 1995 **12**: 73-80.

32. McCord F, Wilson MC. Social problems in geriatric dentistry: an overview. *Gerodontology* 1994 **11**: 63-66.

33. Disability Discrimination Act 1995.

34. Department of Health (1999). Health Survey for England – The Health of Minority Ethnic Groups '99. DoH London.

35. British Dental Association. Improving oral health amongst ethnic minority elderly people. London: BDA, 1996.

36. Griffiths J, Lewis D. Guidelines for the oral care of patients who are dependent, dysphagic or critically ill. *J Disabil Oral Health* 2002 **3**: 30-33.

Chapter 5

Dental services and the dental team

5.1 Introduction

The organisation and availability of dental services varies considerably worldwide. The type of service available, whether private fee-paying, or state subsidised, depends on a number of factors including:

- A country's economic status
- Levels of oral and dental disease
- Political philosophy
- Nature of funding for general health care systems.

In the UK, a general perception of dental services falls into two broad groups, the dentist in 'private practice' and the 'dental hospital service'. There is also some knowledge of particular specialist services, such as oral and maxillo-facial surgery and orthodontics and services for schools and institutions. There have been major changes in the delivery of dental services in the recent decade and changes in the structure of the National Health Service (NHS). This chapter will provide information on the current organisation and functions of dental services, and the current roles of members of the dental team in the countries of the UK. Although it is likely that due to the pace of current legislative change there will be major changes in the delivery of primary dental care[1].

5.2 The history of dentistry

Oral and dental disease has been documented by archaeological studies of the earliest human remains. Evidence of treatment is prehistoric, with the earliest records dating from Egyptian civilisation around 4000 BC. Quite complex treatment was performed in India from 3000 BC. This included extractions, scaling and gingival surgery, and even the transplantation of animal teeth. Diseased teeth and gums were treated by herbs and acupuncture by the Chinese as early as 2000 BC. Extractions are credited to Aesculapius in Greek civilisation in the second century BC. Dentures and bridges made of gold and wired to teeth were worn by the Etruscans around 700 BC.

Hippocrates wrote of health and dental problems around 460 BC. His writings form the basis of the Hippocratic oath to which both doctors and, until recently, dentists pledged themselves upon qualification. Following World War Two and as a result of war crimes against certain races and other groups, a revised code of conduct termed the 'Declaration of Geneva' was introduced to unite members of the medical professions world-wide and to introduce an international code of ethics[2]. This is worth quoting, although a longer declaration now forms the 'International Principles of Ethics for the Dental Profession'.

The Declaration of Geneva

'At the time of being admitted as a member of the Medical Profession, I solemnly pledge myself to consecrate my life to the service of humanity.

I will give to my teachers the respect and gratitude which is their due.

I will practice my profession with conscience and dignity.

The health of my patient will be my first consideration.

I will respect the secrets which are confided in me.

I will maintain by all the means which are in my power the honour and the noble traditions of the medical profession.

My colleagues will be my brothers.

I will not permit considerations of religion, nationality, race, party politics or social standing to intervene between my duty and my patient.

I will maintain the utmost respect for human life from the time of conception: even under threat, I will not use my medical knowledge contrary to the laws of humanity.

I make these promises solemnly, freely and upon my honour.'

Even though the delivery of oral health care has become strongly influenced by commercial and consumerist aspects, the above principles are worth remembering.

By the 4th century, extraction and scaling instruments were available. Although there was some scientific knowledge, dentistry was still surrounded by myth and folklore. Clergymen traditionally carried out healing until the 12th century, until the Pope banned the clergy from performing operations that involved 'blood-letting'. Tooth drawing then moved into the hands of barbers, barber-surgeons, charlatans and even blacksmiths. It was practised in fairs, markets and even on street corners.

Modern dentistry has its origins in the 18th century when Pierre Fouchard, the Surgeon Dentist to Louis XIV, elevated dentistry to a scientific profession. The birth of the profession in the UK took place with the passing of the 1858 Medical Act, followed by the first Dental Act of 1878. It was not until the 1921 Dental Act was passed that dentistry became a closed profession. With the advent of the NHS in 1948 dentistry became freely available to the entire population. Compared with many professions, this makes dentistry a relatively new profession.

5.3 Dental services

Since 1948 there have been many organisational changes in dental services. These have been in response to the changing patterns of oral and dental disease, the socio-political climate and changing perceptions of the value of oral and dental health in society. To enable people to utilise the most appropriate dental service, a brief explanation of the roles and functions of each service is necessary. In the UK there are currently three principal dental services available within the NHS.

- General dental services
- Salaried dental services
- Hospital dental services.

Although this structure has largely been in place since the inception of the NHS, *The Health and Social Care* (*Community Health and Standards*) Act 2003 devolves the responsibility for dental services from central government to Primary Care Trusts (PCTs), with major changes in the way that primary dental care is delivered. This involves local commissioning of dental services and a new approach to contracting with dentists, changing the traditional differences between the general dental services and salaried services. The ways in which dental care is delivered will alter as new guidelines and care pathways are introduced.

5.4 General Dental Services

Most NHS dental care is provided by general dental practitioners and their teams. This is the first choice for routine dental care for most of the population and provides a wide range of preventive and treatment services. Dental care is provided from their own practices, which may also offer a variable range of treatments funded by private health insurance or private fees. All general dental practitioners practising within the NHS are under contract to their local Primary Care Trust (PCT) or equivalent body in Wales, Scotland and Northern Ireland. The PCT holds dental lists, acts as a mediator between the dentist and the public and holds practice information. In the near future they will also hold the funds for NHS dental practice and commission dental care for their local population.

Continuing care

Changes in contracts for general dental practitioners took place in 1990, and patients may now register with a dentist for continuing care in a similar way as with a family doctor[3]. Apart from the obvious advantage of ongoing regular care, registration for continuing care confers other benefits:

- A plan of treatment showing the cost of each item
- Access to emergency out of hours service for advice and treatment
- Free replacement of crowns and fillings less than a year old in certain circumstances.

The continuing care system for adults lapses after fifteen months for adults and one year for children, and patients are encouraged to attend regularly to maintain registration. If the practice is unable, through lack of facilities or expertise, to provide the treatment required, the dentist is obligated to offer a referral to another practice or a specialist practitioner.

Occasional treatment

Occasional treatment, either a single visit or a short course of treatment is also available from general dental practitioners or salaried services providing NHS dental treatment. The full range of more complex treatments like crowns and bridges and the above benefits are not included.

Practice information

To enable the public to make a more informed choice in selecting a dentist suitable for their needs there are a variety of sources of information on the services offered by general dental practices in their locality. Their local PCT or equivalent body will hold information about available practices. Many areas also operate a local dental helpline and co-ordinate access to emergency dental care. Dental practices are also required to produce practice information leaflets. The range of information available includes:

- Normal surgery hours
- Emergency arrangements
- Dentists' qualifications
- Access to premises without the use of stairs
- Access for wheelchair users and other facilities for people with disabilities
- Accessible toilet facilities
- Arrangements for home visits
- In some cases, languages spoken by staff in the practice
- Practice specialities.

Information regarding a person's specific dental problems is also available from NHS Direct, who in some areas, also co-ordinate access to emergency dental care.

Private and NHS treatment

Many general dental practices provide a mixture of dental care under NHS arrangements and private funding arrangements. In the last decade there has been an increase in the number of practices solely providing dental care outside of the NHS contract.

Except for specialist practices, most provide a full range of prevention and treatment. For more complex treatment plans, a system of prior approval is required under NHS arrangements. Advances in dental techniques, dental materials and cosmetic techniques are increasingly offered under privately funded arrangements.

Charges for treatment

In 1948 dental treatment under the NHS was free for everyone. Charges have been introduced over the years, the scale being controlled by government legislation. There is evidence that charges deter patients from seeking care[4]. To encourage attendance Wales has introduced free dental examinations for 18-25 year olds and those aged 65 years and over. Currently, certain items of treatment under the NHS do not carry a patient charge:

- The arrest of haemorrhage
- Re-cementing a bridge
- Repairs to dentures
- An emergency dental call-out or a home visit.

NHS dental treatment is automatically free of patient charges for the following groups:

- Children up to their 18th birthday
- Students in full-time education up to their 19th birthday
- Expectant women and mothers with a baby under one year old
- People receiving certain types of benefits and their spouse or 'partner'
- Holders of exemption certificates.

As the types of benefits and support for people on low income, or with impairments, is under constant change and varies across UK countries it is important that patients seek advice regarding their personal circumstances if they believe they can be supported with dental charges.

For people who are not exempt from dental charges, the current charge (2005) is 80% of the cost of the treatment plan up to a maximum of £354.

The role of the Primary Care Trust\Local Health Board

The PCT, or equivalent body, is responsible for managing and planning family health services in each district. This includes family doctors, dentists, pharmacists and opticians who are contracted to provide NHS care. The devolution of the control of all NHS care to a more local level will have significant implications for NHS dental care. Different systems of funding and delivering dental care are currently being tested which are aimed to improve the distribution of NHS dental services. There is a widespread belief amongst the dental profession and the government that significant changes are required to meet the differing needs of the 21st century.

Overview

The system of continuing care is the mainstay for the General Dental Services. It aims to encourage a partnership between the patient and the dental team and to encourage regular dental attendance to maintain oral health and prevent future oral disease. It places the responsibility for oral health upon the individual, parent or guardian, with the dental team providing support to achieve oral health.

While most general dental practitioners in the UK provide the full range of dental care there has been a growth in the specialised practice providing only certain types of treatment. With the establishment of specialist lists for dentists there are now practices specialising in:

- Orthodontics
- Periodontology
- Implantology
- Endodontics
- Crowns and bridges
- Surgical dentistry.

It is likely that new specialist lists will develop in the near future, including one for special care dentistry.

5.5 Salaried Dental Services

Known also as the Community Dental Service (CDS), it emerged from the School Dental Service. The latter was inspired in the early 20th century by a liberal philosophy to *"educate, nourish and provide health care, including dental care for the semi-literate and poorly fed broad masses of English children"*[5]. It played a major role in taking dental services to children and the most needy, and followed the principles of dental public health in epidemiology and screening for dental disease.

Legislation in 1978 provided new guidelines for the CDS on the inclusion of dental services for the elderly or for disabled people[6]. The development of these services was left to the discretion of health authorities, provided that their obligations to children were met. In 1987 the White Paper *Promoting Better Health*[7] offered further guidance on the development of the CDS with a clear remit to develop dental services for adults with a 'special need'. It provided the service with a commitment to:

- Monitor levels of dental health in all sections of society
- Identify those with special needs
- Organise and provide dental health education
- Provide a safety net for treatment for those whose needs cannot be met by the General Dental Services.

It is proposed that this guidance, issued in 1989, be reviewed. Recent changes in the safety net role have seen the salaried services also provide routine NHS dental care and access to occasional and emergency treatment for those not registered with the General Dental Services.

In practical terms, the Salaried Dental Service complements the General Dental Service in providing dental services to people who are unable to obtain treatment from the latter. The following groups of people are those most likely to receive treatment from the Salaried Services:

- People with learning difficulties
- People with physical impairments
- People with mental health problems
- People with complex medical problems
- Socially disadvantaged
- Geographically isolated
- Communication difficulties
- Frail, impaired older people.

The Salaried Services are well placed to identify needs, initiate new programmes, and expand existing programmes of dental care to 'special care' groups in liaison with General Dental Services and other health care teams. On a practical level, those involved with planning services and packages of care for clients are able to access appropriate dental services for their clients.

Although regular dental care may seem a low priority for many people with special oral health needs, there are advantages in establishing it as opposed to dealing with emergencies. These advantages include, regular assessment, and packages of oral care to prevent oral and dental disease.

Some people will require dental care from specialist centres. It may be more appropriate for them to receive dental care from a mobile facility or in their homes. Close links with hospital-based teams and an outreach approach to care, plus close working with other health care teams will ensure clients are not disadvantaged or discriminated against.

5.6 Hospital Dental Services

The development of the Hospital Dental Services centred on the great seats of medical science in the 19th century. Lectures on dental surgery were given at Guy's Hospital in 1799. In the following year the Royal College of Surgeons received a Royal Charter. Throughout the 19th century dental schools were established and the Royal College of Surgeons held the first examination in dental surgery in 1860. Today, Hospital Dental Services are organised into three areas:

- Dental teaching hospitals
- Oral, dental and maxillo-facial surgery in general hospitals
- Oral and dental services to patients in hospital, mainly those in continuing care.

Dental teaching hospitals

The main responsibility of the teaching hospital and dental school is to train future members of the dental team. Teaching hospitals are part of the university academic system, with consultants in dental specialities employed by the NHS also providing teaching.

Training for dental undergraduates is highly specialised and encompasses a wide range of topics over five years including:

- General medicine and surgery
- Behavioural sciences
- Epidemiology and dental public health
- Oral surgery
- Restorative dentistry
- Paedodontics
- Prevention of oral disease.

Increasingly, teaching is also undertaken on outreach programmes in salaried services' sites. Following graduation there is a further year of vocational training with further training frequently undertaken in the various branches of the dental services. Other members of the dental team are also trained in dental teaching hospitals.

Hospital dental services

Before the Second World War, dental care in provincial hospitals was mainly confined to the extraction of teeth for individuals unable to afford dental care. During the war, maxillo-facial surgery units were established, mainly in military hospitals. This speciality developed, with a new consultant grade established in the 1946 Health Act.

Further specialities appeared later to include the newer dental specialties. These teams, led by consultants accept referrals from medical and dental professionals and often work as part of multi-disciplinary teams in specialist units including, head and neck surgery, plastic surgery and oncology.

5.7 Dental services for in-patients

This service began in 1976 as a response to a lack of organised dental services for patients in continuing care and 'long stay' wards. Since then, changes in patterns of health care have led to a reduced stay in hospitals for many treatments. Many people receive rehabilitation and continuing care in community hospitals, nursing homes and in their own homes. There is still a need, however, for comprehensive routine dental care and many people are at a higher risk of oral and dental disease due to other health problems. Aside from regular care, dental teams working with this client group are often involved in training programmes for nursing teams. Working collaboratively, they are helping to establish nursing standards of care as well as providing dental care in a hospital environment.

5.8 Domiciliary dental care

General dental services and salaried dental services undertake dental care in people's homes and in nursing and residential homes. Mobile dental units and portable equipment are required plus different approaches to dealing with infection control away from the dental surgery.

General dental service

The dental profession has been undertaking domiciliary care for many years, but health care teams and the general public seem unaware that this type of care is available. Details of dental practices providing domiciliary care can be obtained from the Primary Care Trust or equivalent body. For dental care provided under NHS contract the visit itself does not attract a patient charge, however, the usual NHS charges, if applicable, are levied for the dental care provided. With even the most basic of portable equipment a wide range of basic treatments is available including simple restorations, extractions and dentures.

Salaried dental services

In addition to the basic treatments, the use of fully portable dental equipment and mobile dental units, the salaried dental services are able to provide comprehensive care for people unable to access general dental practices. Using the full dental team, preventive packages can also be delivered working closely with the wider health team.

5.9 The dental team

Dentistry has become a specialised profession and the team approach to delivering dental care is being actively developed. The generic term, professionals complementary to dentistry (PCD), covers an expanding team of health workers undertaking specific tasks. In the same way as dentists, PCDs are being registered with the General Dental Council and regulated to ensure admission qualifications, continuing development and a code of practice is followed. Dental team members, although often working independently, work to a treatment plan prescribed by a dentist. The current categories of PCDs are:

- Dental therapists and hygienists
- Dental nurses
- Oral health educators
- Dental technicians.

Dental therapists and hygienists

Although training now produces jointly qualified team members, there was a separate development of the grades. The first training programmes for dental hygienists started in 1913 in the USA against opposition from members of the dental profession. Their role at the time was described as preventing dental disease. Training began in the UK in the armed forces in 1943 and a civilian training programme in 1950. The range of treatments prescribed by dentists was:

- Cleaning and polishing teeth
- Scaling teeth to remove calculus and debris
- Application of certain medicaments
- Application of fluoride and fissure sealants.

Dental hygienists have become established members of the dental team in general dental practice. The joint training programmes and development of the role by the General Dental Council will now see dental therapists and hygienists working in general dental practices. There has been recent expansion of the range of permitted procedures.

Dental therapists began in the UK in 1960. Originally, they were trained to provide basic dental treatment for children and worked in the hospital and community dental services. The range of dental treatment provided included:

- Simple dental fillings
- Extraction of primary teeth
- Cleaning and polishing teeth
- Removal of calculus and scaling of teeth
- Application of certain medicaments
- Application of fluoride and fissure sealants.

Currently, dental therapists have been trained in a more integrated approach with dental undergraduates and gain experience of children's and adult's oral health care.

Dental nurses

Previously known as dental surgery assistants, dental nurses provide support for the operative members of the dental team. Training for the national qualification takes place with commercial training agencies, in general dental practices, salaried dental services and dental teaching hospitals. Their roles include close clinical working, preparation of the dental surgery and infection control. There are additional qualifications available in dental sedation, dental radiography and special care.

Oral health educators

In the more prevention orientated team there is often a member of the dental team to provide oral health education to individuals or small groups. They often have a dental nurse background, with additional qualifications in health education, teaching and communication skills. In the salaried dental services they may be part of a team led by a dental team member with specialised oral health promotion skills working in a multi-agency approach.

Dental technicians

Originally purely based in dental laboratories, dental technicians fabricate dentures, orthodontic appliances, crowns and bridges. There are more specialised technicians who work closely with maxillo-facial teams constructing oral and facial prostheses. There is a proposed new grade of operative dental technician that will also undertake the clinical aspects of denture construction.

Future team roles

As the team approach to dental care develops, other specialist grades will be required, for example, orthodontic therapists to work alongside orthodontic specialists, with expansion of current roles. For dental nurses, there are now additional qualifications to enable them to carry out dental radiography, and in other countries they place fillings and take dental impressions. As many dental practices become larger and as Dental Corporate Bodies (businesses consisting of multiple dental practices) grow, there is a need for trained dental practice managers.

5.10 Future developments in dental care

A number of factors will affect the way in which dental services are delivered in the future, but as with any health care system, funding will determine patterns of care, influenced in turn by the prevailing socio-political ideology. A rising consumerism and more informed dentally aware clients would help to shape future services. Access to the Internet leads to a more informed patient. There is likely to be a more flexible pattern of dental care in terms of when and where dentistry is practised. Increased use of a team approach will mean that the traditional arrangement of the small practice with dentist, dental nurse and receptionist will gradually change and the patient of the future is increasingly likely to be treated by a variety of clinical operators.

As described earlier, there has been a marked improvement in dental health. The reduction in dental caries will reduce the experience of large, multiple fillings. The reduction in periodontal disease will reduce tooth loss and people will remain dentate for their whole lives.

The introduction of clinical governance leads to a dental team that spends more time keeping up to date, undertaking audit and being actively involved in their own continuing education. The use of evidence based protocols will lead to more effective treatment and preventive approaches based on sound research.

New technological developments, particularly in the field of dental materials will continue to drastically alter the way dentistry is carried out. New materials will continue to provide more aesthetic restorations and require less tooth preparation. New techniques of tooth preparation, using lasers and abrasive powders, and chemical materials[8] offer alternative approaches to the rotary instruments currently in use.

Control of pain and discomfort during dental procedures will improve with more profound anaesthesia and electrical fields to block transmissions of pain. Much anxiety and fear of dental treatment can be dealt with effectively by an operator skilled in the techniques of behavioural sciences that are now a part of the undergraduate curriculum.

Even when tooth loss has occurred, there are now alternatives to wearing dentures. Apart from advances in more aesthetic crowns and bridges there will be increased use of dental implants. Many advances in the treatment of periodontal disease have taken place due to greater understanding of the disease process and the use of new materials that encourage regeneration of lost periodontal tissue.

Even though there has been an overall reduction in dental caries levels, it still poses a considerable health problem. Research is continuing into the development of a vaccine against the bacteria in dental plaque that cause dental caries.

In summary, dental surgery and the range of treatments available will continue to develop, coupled with a more effective preventive approach. This will continue to make the dental visit a much less stressful and more comfortable experience and will further lead to more regular dental attendance and a positive impact of oral health.

References

1. Health and Social Care (Community Health and Standards) Bill 2003. www.parliament.uk/bills/bills.cfm
2. Seear J. *Law and ethics in dentistry*. pp113-114. Bristol: Wright, 1981.
3. Central Office of Information. A Change in Dental Care for you. London. HMSO. 1990.
4. Nuttall N, Steele JG, Nunn J *et al.* A guide to the UK Adult Dental Health Survey 1998. p39. London, British Dental Association Publications, 2001.
5. Powell R. The Development and Future Direction of the Community Dental Service in England. Monograph Series. London, University College, University of London. 1988
6. Department of Health and Social Security. Health Circular HC(78)14. London: HMSO, 1978.
7. Promoting Better Health: the Government's Programme for Improving Health Care. Cm 249. London. HMSO. 1987.
8. Maragakis GM, Hahn P, Hellwig E. Chemomechanical caries removal: a comprehensive review of the literature. *Int Dent J* 2001 **51**: 291-299.

Section 2: A guide to oral assessment and oral health care

This section is designed to provide guidance for all health care professionals (and carers) involved in caring for people who need advice, assistance, or support to help meet their daily oral hygiene needs. It is also of relevance to nurse tutors, teachers involved in training dental and other health care professionals, and oral health educators. It is essential reading for people who manage or deliver care across the wide range of health and social care settings in improving the quality oral health care provided and in complying with national guidelines[1-5]. For effective goal setting and individualised care, a clear logical approach is required. The starting point for effective oral care must be an assessment of the individual's needs in order to formulate an appropriate oral care plan.

Although clients themselves can often take part in this assessment process, health professionals are called upon to use their diagnostic skills. Throughout the text there are photographs to illustrate oral conditions in health and disease. Photographs cannot always highlight minor changes of colour and texture in oral tissues. The ability to detect early changes will only develop through training and experience gained by carrying out regular oral examinations. It is recommended that the oral cavity be examined routinely, so that all health care professionals become acquainted with the healthy mouth in all age groups. The authors have noticed that nurses dislike examining mouths and giving oral care in comparison with providing routine care for other parts of the body. Perhaps a period of desensitisation and the information in this text will help to overcome this barrier!

A number of assessment systems are presented so that the most appropriate can be selected. Further research is needed in this area to test and validate criteria. The factors that influence oral health are diverse and complex, nevertheless the basic standards for oral care are fairly universal. Improving the standard of oral care requires a systematic approach encompassing training and resources. So this section contains an action plan for key personnel, for example, the nurse manager, to make it happen. Such a strategy is only likely to succeed with an inter-disciplinary team approach that includes an input from the dental team.

Many oral problems are compounded by medication given for other systemic conditions. An overview of the most common oral side-effects is given but Chapter 8 should not be taken as the only source of information as new drugs with new side-effects are developed.

The tools for oral care are discussed extensively in this section, so that the most effective can be chosen. Nursing research has identified deficiencies in many 'oral toilet' procedures, and practical guidance is offered from a dental perspective. For virtually all oral care procedures, the preferred materials are those the individual would normally use for self-care. Exceptions to this general principle are detailed in Section 3.

References

1. Fiske J, Griffiths J, Jamieson R *et al.* Guidelines for oral health care for long-stay patients and residents. *Gerodontology* 2000 **17**: 55-64.
2. Department of Health. (2001). The essence of care. www.doh.gov.uk/essenceofcare/index/htm
3. Griffiths J. Guidelines for oral health care for people with a physical disability. *J Disabil Oral Health* 2002 **3**: 51-58.
4. Griffiths J, Lewis D. Guidelines for the oral care of patients who are dependent, dysphagic or critically ill. *J Disabil Oral Health* 2002 **3**: 30-33.
5. Welsh Assembly Government. Fundamentals of Care: Guidance for Health and Social Care Staff. 2003.

Chapter 6

Oral assessment

6.1 Introduction

This chapter discusses assessment tools for health professionals in order to facilitate the identification of oral need, risk factors for oral health, the standards and objectives for oral care and formulate an individual oral care plan. Three broad groups of assessment systems are described, those:

- Based on health care professionals, usually nurses, using diagnostic skills to assess changes in the oral cavity
- That are more behavioural, based on observing client's activities
- That involve the client's perceptions of their needs.

Oral assessment is required at key stages during any intervention. It is necessary to identify existing oral needs when the patient or client is seen at the commencement of a period of care. This increases the likelihood of early detection of treatable oral disease, and appropriate pharmacological interventions and further referral[1]. The oral care needs of a dependent person also require monitoring during the presenting or acute phase of illness and subsequently at agreed intervals during rehabilitation and recovery.

No single assessment system [currently available] meets all the criteria; indeed, considering the diversity of the oral needs of different client groups, it is unlikely that one system could meet all requirements. It is encouraging to see the increasing number of well researched and evidence based papers in the nursing press that refer to the importance of carrying out an oral assessment[2-11]. A review of some assessments reported in the literature is provided together with those currently used by the authors. Most systems will require to be tailored to specific locations if they are to be sensitive to the needs of specific client groups. Colour illustrations will assist in learning to assess oral conditions and make comparisons between healthy and unhealthy or diseased mouths.

6.2 Types of oral need

Oral and dental needs can be classified into three commonly used descriptions used for health needs:

- Normative need
- Felt need
- Expressed need.

Normative need is the need as defined by health professionals. Felt and expressed needs are those defined by the client. Normative need is consistently higher than clients' felt or expressed needs. This has lead to a difference in fulfilling those needs, with only the tip of a 'clinical iceberg' having their needs met by health services. Unmet needs have been shown for all age groups in epidemiological surveys; for example, the level of untreated dental caries in children's teeth[12] and also in adults in the UK[13].

The most important point for health professionals to remember is that they will encounter unmet oral and dental needs in someone presenting with other health problems. These needs will impinge on and affect the individual's general health status and should be addressed. In fact addressing those needs may even play a part in the rehabilitation process. For example, there is increasing evidence to suggest that the bacteria involved in periodontal disease are associated with aspiration infections and poor glycemic control in Type II diabetes[14].

Maintenance of good oral hygiene may reduce oral and pharyngeal colonisation by potential respiratory pathogens[15] and help reduce the incidence of these potentially life-threatening diseases. Research in these areas is continuing and may provide a better insight into the relationship between oral and systemic health.

6.3 Key indicators requiring assessment

The key areas that will give an indication of oral health status and point towards objectives for care include:

- The presence of existing symptoms and signs of oro-dental disease including early changes to dental and soft tissues
- Current mouth care practices and preventive behaviour, including patterns of dental service attendance
- The presence of risk factors including systemic disease, medication and/or impairment
- The presence of key stressors for oral health.

These areas provide the basis for assessment tools that weigh the different factors, quantify risk status, and can be subsequently translated into the degree and type of intervention required.

6.4 Current reported oral assessment systems

Most oral assessment systems have been developed to monitor changes in oral tissues in response to systemic disease or to evaluate nursing interventions. They are mainly diagnostic in approach and tend to be restricted to high risk groups. The effects of radiotherapy and chemotherapy on oral health status are serious and potentially life threatening, particularly for children. The need for accurate baseline information to allow rapid changes to be measured has been stressed. Many of the assessment tools have therefore been based on the earlier work of Eilers *et al.*[16] who developed a very reliable assessment tool for use in oncology. It includes assessment of the voice and the ability to swallow, important areas for assessment during the various stages of treatment involving radiotherapy, chemotherapy and bone marrow transplants.

Nursing assessments have since been developed for patients with advanced cancer[9] and patients in intensive care[17]. However, standards of oral care have been identified to be inadequate in other areas of nursing care[18]. A wide gap between theory and practice is reported[19] with curricular deficiencies in pre and post registration nurse training in oral care[20,21] and a lack of training in residential care facilities[22]. Since the first edition of this book there has been greater awareness of the need for improved standards of oral care across all care settings. This has been reflected in national guidance that recommends individual oral assessment and improved standards of oral care based on clinical effectiveness[23,24].

Assessment tools have been developed for in-patients[2], older dependent patients[8,25,] psychiatric patients[26] and people with Alzheimer's disease[27]. Oral assessment based on the Royal College of Surgeons guidelines for the oral management of oncology patients requiring radiotherapy, chemotherapy and bone marrow transplantation contains an oral assessment guide adapted from Eilers *et al.*[16] and detailed protocols for intervention before, during and after cancer therapy[28,29] (Chapter 18, *Tables 18.5-18.7*). This assessment is used by the Host Defence Unit at Great Ormond Street Hospital. An oral assessment guide and protocol for care of patients who are dependent, dysphagic or critically ill[30] is reproduced in Chapter 18 (Table 18.6).

Most assessment tools record the appearance of hard and soft tissues of the mouth and associated structures, the appearance and consistency of saliva, and oral odour[8], while others also include assessment of voice and swallow[29]. Numerical recording systems do not always correlate with the patient's oral care needs. It is interesting to note that as the result of an audit into mouth care in cancer nursing, scoring has been removed because it did not reflect individual patient's needs[31]. Without intensive training and calibration of all staff carrying out the assessment, there is likely to be variation between assessors. The scoring system based on RCS guidelines is used as a guide for dental referral rather than for a specific oral intervention[29]. Increasingly, oral assessment tools are being developed in collaboration with the dental team and designed to be specific to the client group being assessed. This is a very welcome development in inter-disciplinary care.

6.5 Assessment based on observed and reported behaviour

While most hospital-based systems are designed for nurses and health professionals to make an assessment using their clinical expertise, there is also a place for the behavioural approach. If the patient or client's behaviour is measured against a set of objectives over a period of time, a more reliable indicator of dependence can be determined. This type of system is more appropriate during rehabilitation or in a continuing care setting when long-term care and coping strategies are being assessed and developed. At this stage, wider involvement of other members of the health care team and carers requires an assessment process that is not based on clinical expertise.

Since many factors may directly or indirectly affect a person's ability to maintain oral health, other indicators may be included to assess the level of intervention required. An oral risk assessment that includes stressors for oral health, designed to be incorporated into specific assessment systems for different client groups was successfully piloted in a neuro-psychiatry unit for adults with acquired brain injury, predominantly younger males[32]. This is a Joint Educational Nursing Assessment Tool designed for collaborative oral health care. It acts as a nursing risk assessment and informed referral. It permits the dental team to highlight the oral side-effects of medication and provide feed back for an interim care plan until the patient receives a detailed oral examination by a dentist. The assessment has been adapted and is used in a challenging behaviour unit for adults with a learning disability, in a stroke rehabilitation unit, rehabilitation for acquired brain injuries, rehabilitation and continuing care of older people and the elderly mentally ill *(Table 6.1)*.

Whichever assessment is used, initial training must be given. The amount of time needed to carry out an assessment will vary. To facilitate reporting and monitoring, details of any oral abnormalities may be recorded on an oral chart *(Figure 6.1)*.

6.6 Assessment involving the client's views

The assessment of oro-dental needs involving clients themselves has an important role in obtaining a more accurate appreciation of felt and

Table 6.1 Joint Assessment Nursing Education Tool (JANET)

Name _____	**Status** Day ☐	Respite ☐
Address: _____	Acute ☐	Cont Care ☐
	Rehab ☐	Comm Care ☐

Status Day ☐ Respite ☐
Acute ☐ Cont Care ☐
Rehab ☐ Comm Care ☐

Impairment:
Physical ☐ Cognitive ☐
Mental health ☐ Learning diff ☐
Communication ☐ Other ☐

Name _____
Address: _____

DOB: _____ **ID No:** _____

Date of admission: _____

Date of discharge: _____

Mobility: Ambulant ☐
Needs assistance ☐
Wheelchair user ☐
Bedfast ☐
Hoist transfer ☐

ASSESSMENT	INTERIM CARE PLAN
Natural teeth: Yes ☐ No ☐ D/Know ☐ Number if known and appearance Comments:	
Dentures Yes ☐ No ☐ D/Know ☐ Full upper ☐ Partial upper ☐ Full lower ☐ Partial lower ☐ Worn regularly Yes ☐ No ☐ Worn at night Yes ☐ No ☐ Labelled Yes ☐ No ☐ Denture Hygene Good ☐ Poor ☐ Appearance Broken ☐ Cracked ☐ Rough ☐ Stained ☐ Comments:	
Complaints Yes ☐ No ☐ D/Know ☐ Teeth ☐ Gums ☐ Denture ☐ Other ☐ Specify: Pain ☐ Swelling ☐ Halitosis ☐ Bleeding Gums ☐ Difficulty eating ☐ Loose Dentures ☐ Dry mouth ☐ Comments:	
Habits / Lifestyle: eg diet, sugar intake, smoking, alchohol, drugs, Pica etc	

ASSESSMENT	INTERIM CARE PLAN
Diet Normal ☐　Soft ☐　　Puree ☐ NG ☐　PEG ☐　　Special ☐ Thickened ☐　Food supplements ☐ Comments:	
Stressors for oral health Level of hydration ☐　O² therapy ☐ Medical problems ☐　Tracheotomy ☐ Facial weakness/paralysis ☐　Cleft palate ☐ Risk of aspiration ☐　Dysphagia ☐ Challenging behaviour ☐　Epilepsy ☐ Mouth breathing ☐　Trismus ☐ Comments:	
Prescribed medication: Yes ☐　　No ☐ Record whether liquid, tablet, IM, IV or other _____ _____ _____ _____ _____ _____ _____ _____ _____ _____ _____	
Manual disability:　Yes ☐　No ☐ Change in use of dominant hand: Yes ☐　No ☐	
Dental attendance: Dental appointment in the last year: Yes ☐　No ☐　D/know ☐ Record name and address of dentist if known	

Completed by: _____ Status _____ Date _____

Address: _____ Tel: _____

FORWARD COMPLETED ASSESSMENT TO: _____

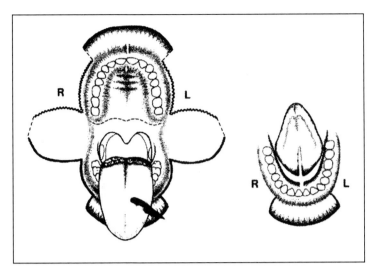

Figure 6.1 To facilitate reporting and monitoring, details of any oral abnormalities may be recorded on an oral chart

expressed needs. Although undoubtedly there is a gap between the provision of normative need (as assessed by the dental profession) and perceived need (as articulated by the client), it is difficult to assess how much of this gap is due to an inappropriate assessment of normative needs.

Hoad-Reddick[33] reviewed the differences between perceived need and normative need in a wide cross-section of studies; the difference ranged between 12-49%. It is axiomatic that any measurement of need which includes the views of the client is likely to be more sensitive. In this study, the need for treatment was assessed by a list of questions:

- Do you think you need any dental treatment?
- What type of treatment is needed?
- Do you have any painful areas in your mouth?
- Do you have any problems eating?
- When did you last visit a dentist?
- How old are your dentures?

A simple visual examination by care workers was found to correlate closely with the need for treatment as assessed by a dental professional. This concept was developed to assess the potential needs of older people attending a rehabilitation day unit and further developed to include other risk factors such as smoking and medication with possible oral side-effects[34] (*Table 6.2*). It provides a simple mechanism for opportunistic

Table 6.2

ORAL HEALTH RISK ASSESSMENT[34]

Oral health assessment by health professionals provides a mechanism for opportunistic identification of clients who have oral and/or dental problems, are not receiving regular dental care and/or are at risk of poor oral health. Subjective indicators include the ability to speak, smile or eat without pain or discomfort. This example of an Oral Health Assessment may be adapted to suit any client group or adapted for self assessment. It is recommended that risk assessments are used in collaboration with local dental services in order to facilitate access to an appropriate dental service. The Community Dental Service is best placed to fulfil the role of facilitator. **A response in a highlighted area signifies a need for further investigation or action.**

1. Does the client have natural teeth?	❏ NO	❏ YES	❏ Don't Know
2. Does the client wear dentures?	❏ NO	❏ YES Specify ❏ Upper ❏ Lower	❏ Don't Know
a) If YES, are dentures labelled?	❏ YES	❏ NO	❏ Don't Know
b) If YES, how old are dentures?	❏ > 5 yrs	❏ < 5yrs	❏ Don't Know
3. Does the client have any problems? eg pain, discomfort, difficulty eating, decayed teeth, denture problems, ulcers, dry mouth, halitosis etc. **If YES, describe the problem.**	❏ NO	❏ YES	❏ Don't Know
4. Does the client smoke or have a past history of smoking?	❏ NO	❏ YES	❏ Don't Know
5. Is the client taking medication? **Check the British National Formulary for any oral side-effects**	❏ NO	❏ YES	❏ Don't Know
6. Is urgent dental treatment required?	❏ NO	❏ YES	❏ Don't Know
7. Date of last dental treatment?	❏ > 1yr	❏ < 1 yr	❏ Don't Know
8. Registered for dental care? If Yes, record name and address of dentist.	❏ YES	❏ NO	❏ Don't Know

Adapted from Griffiths[37]. Reproduced with kind permission of Professor June Nunn, Editor, *Journal of Disability and Oral Health* identification of clients who have oral problems, identifies risk factors for oral health and clients who not receiving regular dental care. A response in a highlighted area signifies a need for further action.

6.7 The self-caring individual

For people who are hospitalised or in residential care, their very presence indicates a state of dependence, however temporary. Support for oral care in hospital and nursing homes has also been demonstrated to be inadequate[18,35]. It is documented that in long term care facilities, numerous problems mitigate against routine provision of oral health care and encourage neglect[36]. Some of the reasons for neglect include:

- Care staff placing patients' dental care as a low priority
- Long term care staff limitations
- Heavy work loads and more pressing tasks to perform
- Chronic inadequate oral hygiene practices.

Mandatory staff training in oral care is a major issue within this sector. Guidelines for the development of local standards of oral health care address these issues[36]. If the individual is self-caring with respect to their oral health, the role of health professionals and care providers is to ensure that they have access to the necessary equipment and facilities summarised below and the required level of support to sustain self-care:

Mouth and tooth cleaning equipment

- Toothbrush and toothpaste
- Dental floss or other interdental cleaners
- Denture brush and denture cleaner

Access to suitable facilities

- Suitable privacy
- Clean running water
- Mirror at an appropriate height or position
- Glass or receptacle for rinsing
- Container for storage of dentures and other appliances or prostheses

Access to appropriate information and advice
- Information regarding facilities

- Dental services available
- Appropriate preventive advice.

6.8 The dependent individual

The degree of individual dependence will vary and in response to the patient's systemic condition. However when oral care has to be undertaken by a health professional, i.e. the patient is totally dependent for oral needs, procedures in Chapter 18 should be followed (*Tables 18.5, 18.6*). Gloves should be worn for all procedures involving contact with oral tissues and for handling dentures.

6.9 Summary

Three types of assessment systems are described. The first is based on documenting the presence of existing signs and symptoms of oral disease including early changes to hard and soft tissues in the oral cavity by nurses or other health professionals, and is mainly used for the dependent patient. In addition to changes in the mouth, other risk factors for oral health are identified. Examples in the nursing and dental literature are reviewed. The second type of assessment is behavioural and based on what clients can do. These systems can be used in a multi-disciplinary context as the outcomes may involve different health professionals working together. The third type of assessment involves the client's own perception of their oro-dental needs. A series of oral care procedures are also covered in Chapters 2, 16 and 18.

All health professionals have a code of professional conduct that covers their responsibility to act in the best interests of the patient. Caring for the mouth is recognised as one of the most basic nursing activities. It is essential therefore that an appropriate oral assessment is used to identify individual needs and therefore the most appropriate oral hygiene interventions. This principle should apply not only to the nursing profession but across all care settings for people who are dependent on others for the daily care needs.

References

1. Sweeney MP. Mouth care in nursing. Part 3: Oral care for the dependent patient. *J Nurs Care* 1998 Autumn: 7 – 9.

2. Rattenbury N, Mooney G, Bowen J. Oral assessment and care for in-patients. *Nurs Times* 1999 49: 52-53.

3. Xavier G. The importance of mouth care in preventing infection. *Nursing Standard* 2000 14: 47-51.

4. Freer SK. Use of an oral assessment tool to improve practice. *Prof Nurs* 2000 15: 635-637.

5. Roberts J. Developing an oral assessment and intervention tool for older people: 1. *Br J Nursing* 2000 9: 1124-1127.

6. McNeill HE. Biting back at poor oral hygiene. *Intensive Crit Care Nurs* 2000 16: 367-372.

7. Rawlins CA, Trueman IW. Effective mouth care for seriously ill patients. *Prof Nurs* 2001 16: 1025-1028.

8. Dickinson H, Watkins C, Leathley M. The development of the THROAT: the holistic and reliable oral assessment tool. *Clin Effectiveness in Nursing* 2001 5: 104-110.

9. Milligan S, McGill M, Sweeney MP *et al.* Oral care for people with advanced cancer: an evidence based protocol. *Int J Pall Nurs* 2001 7: 418-427.

10. Lee L, White V, Ball J *et al.* An audit of oral care practice and staff knowledge in hospital palliative care. *Int J Pall Nurs* 2001 7: 395-400.

11. Clay M. Nelson D. Assessing oral health in older people. *Nursing Older People* 2002 14: 31-32.

12. Pitts NB, Boyles J, Nugent ZJ *et al.* The dental caries experience of 5 year-old children in England and Wales. Surveys co-ordinated by the British Association for the Study of Community Dentistry 2001/2002. *Community Dent Health* 2003 30: 45-54.

13. Nuttal N, Steele JG, Pine C *et al.* A Guide to the UK Adult Dental Health Survey 1998. London: British Dental Association, 2001.

14. Taylor GW, Loesche WJ, Terpenning MS. Impact of oral disease on systemic health in the elderly: diabetes mellitus and aspiration pneumonia. *J Pub Health Dent* 2000 60: 313-320.

15. Imsand M, Janssens J-P, Auckenthaler R et al. Bronchopneumonia and oral health in hospitalised older patients. A pilot study. *Gerodontology* 2002 19: 66-72.

16. Eilers J. Berger A, Peterson M. Development, testing and application of the Oral Assessment Guide. *Oncol Nurs Forum* 1988 15: 325-330.

17. Jenkins D. Oral care in ICU: an important nursing role. *Nurs Stand* 1989 4: 24-28.

18. Longhurst R. An evaluation of the oral care given to patients when staying in hospital. *Primary Dent Care* 1999 6: 112-115

19. Wilkin K. A critical analysis of the philosophy, knowledge and theory underpinning mouth care practice for the intensive care unit. *Intensive Crit Care Nurs* 2002 18: 181-188.

20. Longhurst R. A cross-sectional study of the oral health care instruction given to nurses during their basic training. *Br Dent J* 1998 **184**: 453-457.

21. White R. Nurse assessment of oral health: a review of practice and education. *Br J Nurs* 2000 **9**: 260-266.

22. Frenkel H. Behind the screens: care staff observations on delivery of oral health care in nursing homes. *Gerodontology* 1999 **16**: 75-80.

23. Department of Health. (2001). The essence of care. www.doh.gov.uk/essenceofcare/index/htm

24. Welsh Assembly Government. Fundamentals of Care: Guidance for Health and Social Care Staff. 2003.

25. Roberts J. Developing an oral assessment and intervention tool for older people: 3. *Br J Nursing* 2000 **9**: 2073-2078.

26. Sjogren R, Nordenstrom G. Oral health status of psychiatric patients. *J Clin Nurs* 2000 **9**: 632-638.

27. Lin CY, Jones DB, Godwin K *et al.* Oral health assessment by nursing staff of Alzheimer's patients in a long-term-care facility. *Spec Care Dent* 1999 **19**: 64-71.

28. Royal College of Surgeons of England. Dental Faculty. 2001. www.rcseng.ac.uk

29. Fiske J, Lewis D. Guidelines for the oral management of oncology patients requiring radiotherapy, chemotherapy and bone marrow transplantation. Report of BSDH Working Group. *J Disab Oral Health* 2001 **2**: 3-14.

30. Griffiths J, Lewis D. Guidelines for the oral care of patients who are dependent, dysphagic or critically ill. *J Disabil Oral Health* 2002 **3**: 30-33.

31. Honnor A, Law A. Mouth care in cancer nursing: using an audit to change practice. *Br J Nurs* 2002 **11**: 1087-1096.

32. Griffiths JE, Williams J. Risk factors for oral health in neuro-psychiatric patients in a rehabilitation unit. Japanese Society of Dentistry for the Handicapped. Abstracts / Proceedings. Supp. 1998 **19**: 347.

33. Hoad-Reddick G. A study to determine oral health needs of institutionalised elderly patients by non-dental health care workers. *Community Dent Oral Epidemiol* 1991 **19**: 233-236.

34. Griffiths J. Guidelines for oral health care for people with a physical disability. *J Disabil Oral Health* 2002 **3**: 51-58.

35. Frenkel H, Harvey I, Newcombe RG. Oral health among nursing home residents in Avon. *Gerodontology* 2000 **17**: 33-38.

36. Fiske J, Griffiths J, Jamieson R *et al.* Guidelines for oral health care for long-stay patients and residents. *Gerodontology* 2000 **17**: 55-64.

37. Griffiths JE. An oral health assessment carried out by nurses to identify older people needing advice and support in accessing dental services. *In* Knook DL *et al.* 1995. Ageing in a changing Europe: Abstracts III European Congress of Gerontology (Abst No 026.0807).

Chapter 7

The role of nursing and care managers in promoting oral care

7

7.1 Introduction

The role of the Nurse Manager and Care Manager at ward or community level is pivotal in making things happen. It is essential that the whole issue of oral care is addressed at this level to ensure that the different activities and professions are brought together to maintain a high standard of oral care at the interface with the patient or client. This chapter applies equally to care managers working in the private and voluntary care sectors, and in the provision of community care. It is the nursing or care team, led by its manager which has intimate knowledge of an individual patient or client's needs, and which is responsible for continuing rather than episodic care. The Government has taken action to improve standards of care in care homes through a new National Care Standards Commission and through the Better Care, Higher Standards charters[1]. Clear and specific recommendations to improve standards of oral care are given in *Essence of Care* and *Fundamentals of Care*[2,3]. This chapter is designed to help managers to comply with the guidance and assist oral health educators in establishing appropriate training programmes.

Good oral care is more than ensuring adequate access to dental professionals for treatment, even though this baseline level of service is difficult enough to obtain in many areas of health care. Older people and those with dementia experience particular problems accessing NHS dental care[4]. Older people in residential care do not receive uniformly high standards of oral health care and physical access to dental services is also a problem[5-7]. Care staff criticise management's lack of arrangements for routine dental examination, lack of commitment to staff training and lack of provision of necessary oral hygiene equipment for residents[8].

Although oral health care may not be the primary reason for the initial referral for nursing care, unmet oral needs are found in many groups of patients and client groups. Those needs may not have been expressed, and a strategy is required to examine oral health needs and to provide the mechanism to meet them. This applies not just to the period of nursing care, but also to helping to support individual coping strategies to maintain oral health in all care supported environments. This chapter sets out the areas of an effective oral health strategy that will enable compliance with national guidelines, and then discusses the practical contents of such programmes.

7.2 Development of an oral health strategy

An effective oral health strategy will contain several key elements. These

Table 7.1 Nursing standards for oral health in continuing care[9]

Standards for oral health must address:	Needs of residents / clients Knowledge Environment Equipment Oral hygiene practices Resources

STANDARD

Residents will have equal opportunity for good oral health as the self-caring individual.

STRUCTURE

All nurses and health care professionals will have a basic knowledge and understanding of the importance of oral health and disease.
Oral assessment will be used to identify oral status and oral hygiene needs.
There will be a clear referral procedure for routine and emergency dental advice and treatment.
Oral hygiene equipment appropriate to a resident's needs will be available.

Standard equipment will include:	Tooth brushes Toothpaste Denture brush Denture bowl

Specific oral hygiene aids recommended by the dental team will be available.
Residents will have access to privacy for oral hygiene.
Information will be available for residents and staff.

PROCESS

A baseline oral assessment will be carried out to identify the resident's oral status and risk factors for oral health.
After assessment, the resident will be provided with oral hygiene equipment appropriate to their needs.
Oral assessment will be repeated at specified intervals to monitor the effectiveness of oral care.
Oral care will be carried out as specified according to the resident's needs.
Staff will support, motivate and assist residents to carry out oral care.

OUTCOME

Identified oral care plan for resident's needs.
Provision of appropriate oral hygiene equipment and regular assessment will seek to maintain and prevent deterioration in the resident's oral status.
To maintain oral health, enhance oral comfort, prevent oral disease and handicap.

Fiske *et al* (2000)[9]. Reproduced with kind permission of Dr James Newton, Editor, *Gerodontology*.

include the use of effective oral assessment criteria at the start of care because many client groups, for example older people and people with a learning difficulty have lower perceived and expressed oral needs. Chapter 6 describes some of the current criteria used. However it is important that these criteria are linked to nursing objectives. Key elements of an oral health strategy include:

- Oral assessment at the first point of contact
- Environmental factors
- Access to oral hygiene equipment
- Staff Training
- Access to dental service.

BSDH Guidelines give examples of standards for oral health in residential care settings[9]. An example of agreed nursing standards for oral health in a continuing care ward for adults with profound learning disability is reproduced in *Table 7.1*. These can be adapted to suit other client groups in a range of care settings[9].

7.3 Continuing education and training

Oral care has a low status in the present training of nurses[10,11] In the private and voluntary sectors where care staff may have a social care rather than health care background and where there is a high staff turnover, training has a lower status. Standards of mouth care in professional settings have been demonstrated to be inadequate and based on inappropriate tools and materials[9,10,12-15]. Even within high risk groups such as children receiving cancer treatments, oral care protocols are inconsistent and inadequate[16].

It is important to address the continuing education needs of all staff grades involved in personal care. As nursing care is increasingly provided by a team approach, it is vital that all team members receive training and education, particularly the non-professionally trained who are more likely to be involved with meeting the needs of people with a high level of dependency. For example, the effect of an oral health education programme on participants' attitudes towards oral health persisted for at least three years; this study suggested that trainees with a low level of health care education benefited most[17].

Training for these groups is particularly important because, as with any task-orientated group, their original training may have lacked the conceptual understanding of the need for oral care. For example, staff employed to provide care and support for people with a learning disability living in the

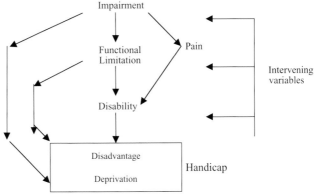

This concept is based on the medical model of disability (WHO 1980)

Impairment:	Anatomical loss, structural abnormality or disturbance in biochemical or physiological processes which arise as a result of disease or injury or is present at birth
Functional limitation:	Restrictions in the functions customarily expected of the body or its component organs or systems
Pain and discomfort:	Self-reported pain and discomfort, physical and psychological symptoms and other not directly observable feelings, states or manifestations which impinge on the individual or others
Disability:	Any limitation in or lack of ability to perform the activities of daily living
Handicap:	The disadvantage and deprivation experienced by people with impairments, functional limitations, pain and discomfort or disabilities because they cannot or do not conform to the expectations of the groups to which they belong

Figure 7.1 The impact of oral disorders: a conceptual framework. Locker [18] Reproduced with the kind permission of Professor Denis O'Mullane, Editor, Community Dental Health

community receive mandatory training in administering medication, dealing with epilepsy and CPR, but training in oral care is patchy and not mandatory even though the outcome of poor or inadequate oral care may result in a crisis need for treatment under general anaesthesia. Even though the professionally trained nurse may have completed an oral assessment for a patient and set care goals, health care support workers may not have the skills to implement the tasks. This may seem obvious, but it is easy to overlook the fact that our personal care skills are not always appropriate for those in our care, and that specialist approaches may be needed.

The importance of continuing education to provide a regular update of oral needs is becoming increasingly apparent both within the dental profession and in the wider health professions. Changes in oral health status will mean that client groups will have different oral health needs to those of their stereotypical portrayal. For example, increasing numbers of older people are retaining teeth into later life in most industrialised countries.

Specific risk groups for oral and dental disease are emerging. Most available research data on oral care carried out by nurses has been obtained from studies on patients with cancer or those in intensive care units (Chapter 6). This may be because in those specified areas, oral care is more problematic and deficiencies in oral care produce overt problems e.g. mucositis. For many client groups in nursing care, whether continuing or short term, oral care is a quality of life issue[18,19]. Although based on the medical model of disability (a concept which is not accepted by the disability movement), Locker's conceptual framework of the impact of oral disorders gives an insight into the potential impact of oral problems on quality of life (*Figure 7.1*)[18].

Methods of providing oral care, the most appropriate tools, and the degree of oral care required are issues that need to be addressed[15]. Nursing research identifies the inadequate scientific basis of many existing procedures[14,20-25]. Care and security of dentures is also inadequate because staff lack adequate information on the subect[8,12,26,27].

One of the primary aims of this book is to provide a core of knowledge for use in continuing education and training; the first section provided the basic knowledge and skills needed, while Section 3 highlights the specific needs of different client groups.

7.4 A ward or community based programme: a case for oral care

The implementation of hospital-based, organisational-based or district-based policies and guidelines at a field level is a task clearly within the remit of the manager. It is fair to state that there are few areas of care in which there are not many competing pressures for time and resources. This is a situation that is unlikely to change in the future, as demographic changes in most industrialised societies tend towards an ageing population presenting greater demands. However, effective oral care need not be time-consuming. Certainly where it is practised in a 'hands-on' manner, it can be made more effective without increasing the time needed. The manager is in the position of being able to balance the needs of the client group with the individual's needs and with the rationing of staff and non-staff resources. The likely outcomes of an effective oral assessment will be in three main areas:

- A health promotion need for the nurse / carer to help the individual develop more effective oral self-care skills
- A need for assistance with oral care in the short or long term for

individuals with a degree of dependence to meet their daily needs

- A treatment need requiring the intervention of the dental profession.

7.5 The interdisciplinary approach

The compartmentalised approach to the delivery of health care in most countries means that many members of the health care team work in isolation of each other, and that interdisciplinary co-operation exists in theory rather than practice. For example, drooling often attributed to excessive salivation is a problem that can seriously influence social acceptance. Patients may be prescribed hyoscine to reduce salivation. However in many cases, particularly for example in Parkinson's disease, the problem is generally not due to hyper-salivation, but to posture and delayed swallow. The intended reduction in saliva by prescribing hyoscine may have a detrimental effect on the oral tissues. However, the input of a physiotherapist to improve posture may be more beneficial in reducing drooling.

The primary health care approach has been one solution, but in any organisation there are a number of key people employed to bring others together. The nurse manager for example is placed in a position to control the whole process (*Figure 7.2*).

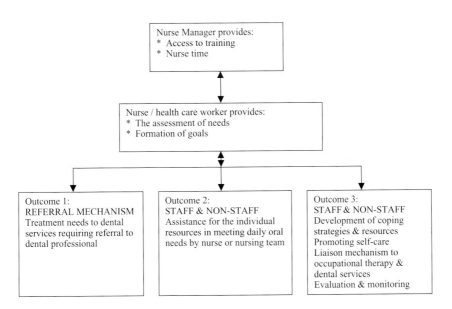

Figure 7.2 The individual with oral needs

7.6 Keeping the issue of oral care on the agenda

The evaluation and revisiting of individual objectives in care plans will note the changes in status of the patient as he or she moves through the process of treatment to rehabilitation and recovery.

This will be accompanied by changes in oral status and oral needs as drug therapy changes and the individual becomes more self-reliant or develops coping skills. An efficient referral mechanism is required as the changes in oral status may necessitate interventions by the dental team. An example of a referral is given in Chapter 6 *(Table 6.1)*.

7.7 Putting the strategy into action: providing the training

Whichever oral assessment procedure is selected as being most appropriate, it is likely that there will be a training need to ensure that all staff are conversant with its use. Sufficient research into current nurse-based oral and mouth-care practices has been done to show that many existing procedures are outdated, ineffective and based on non-empirical findings[15]. It is argued that one of the fundamental reasons for this is nursing dependence on the medical profession as its source of knowledge and focus for practice[28]. However doctors have little knowledge about dental problems[29]. In the authors' experience, working primarily within the hospital sector, medical staff generally have little knowledge of oral disease or the possible impact of the side-effects of medication on oral health.

Perhaps another reason for many of these shortcomings lies in poor communication within the dental profession, which has failed to involve itself sufficiently in the formulation and review of procedures. Despite a challenge to the dental profession to be involved in training from several seminal nurse-based research articles, there have been only a few reported programmes in which there has been close co-operation between the nursing and dental professions in training and devising programmes[10,30]. The massive growth in the care sector that has developed with the concept of community care will generate an even greater need for training programmes.

Staff training programmes have tended to focus on the student's personal oral skills. The rationale behind this approach was that improvement of personal oral practices would lead to greater competency in the oral care of clients. But since the practice of effective oral care requires modification of care to the client's needs, it is questionable whether this approach is appropriate as it may not encourage objectivity in assessment. Furthermore, when newly qualified staff encounter out-moded oral practices, there may be reluctance to implement their new knowledge and skill. A change in the philosophy of care with regard to oral care is required in order to promote changes in practice. However, it does provide an excellent starting point, and if appropriately handled, can help to minimise some of the barriers and negative views that mouth care seems to produce among nurses.

7.8 Meeting the training needs of the whole team

When training needs are being reviewed, the needs of night staff and shift workers should be considered and programmes timetabled to address this problem.

The specialist content for training can be obtained from the dental team, but the manager should specify training needs very clearly so that the programme is oriented to the client group being cared for. It will be a more efficient use of training resources if nurse trainers themselves undergo this oral training so that the knowledge and skills acquired can be 'cascaded' throughout the team. With the current national shortage of nurses and health care workers, and the difficulty in releasing staff for training, the appointment of a link nurse trained in oral care appropriate to clients' needs with responsibility for oral care and local training has been demonstrated to be an effective and successful use of resources[31,32]. It is essential that members of the dental team with expertise in the specific areas of care being addressed are involved in developing the content of the training programme or providing the initial training.

As with all practical skills, adequate provision for hands-on training is essential, and in the learning environment, the group itself can provide this opportunity by practising on each other's mouths. The dental hygienist is the key member of the team with regard to the practical aspects of mouth care.

7.9 What to include in the training programme

The content of a training programme should be tailored to meet the oral health issues of the specific client group. However, there will be a common core component. We suggest that the core knowledge as found in Chapter 2 is an essential starting point, followed by the sections that are relevant to the particular client group. It is worth noting that most adults will already feel that they have a reasonable level of competency in personal oral practices and will need opportunities for practice and consideration before adapting. A small group approach that allows students to explore their own dental opinions, and their views and anxieties about oral care or handling dentures is likely to be more successful.

Table 7.2 Curriculum Content for Nurse Training[30]

A holistic approach based on The Scientific Basis of Oral Health and Disease

Objectives: Provide a basic understanding of

Periodontal disease

Dental Caries

Role of saliva

Oral infections

Oral cancers

Oral side of effects of medication

Basic messages for prevention

Oral hygiene techniques and materials

Care of dentures

The curriculum content for a common foundation programme is based on the needs of the self-caring individual.

Teaching throughout other branches of nursing would reflect the particular oral health issues of specific client groups, for example:

Care of Children

Care of Older People

Learning Disabilities

Mental Health Problems

Medically Compromised

Intensive Care

Malignant Disease

Infectious Diseases

Dysphagia

Palliative Care.

Modules are adapted to specific conditions eg care of children with malignant disease, stroke, multiple sclerosis or Parkinson's disease for post-qualification training programmes.

It is also suggested that the oral needs of the client group be covered in a separate session to highlight the modifications and special approaches that may be needed. For example, Learning Disability Guidelines highlight the management of specific complications that may affect people with a learning disability[33]. These topics should be included in the specialised component of training for health care professionals for this client group. Boyle describes the content of the core curriculum first developed for Project 2000 nurse training (*Table 7.2*) which was subsequently adapted for pre and post-qualification nurse training[30].

7.10 Resources at ward or community level for self-care

The requirements at ward or community level will be moderated by the needs of the client group and the degree of oral self-care encountered. Except for the very few patients who are totally dependent, patients will themselves be involved in the care of their own mouths.

There are a number of central requirements that the manager can ensure are met in order to minimise barriers to oral care. These include the physical requirements of access to:

- Clean, preferably running water and access to a sink or alternative
- A suitable mirror and adequate illumination
- Appropriate equipment: toothbrushes, denture brushes, cleaning pastes, dental floss, inter-dental brushes, and any aids or modifications to meet the individual's needs
- Dental services for screening and treatment.

Other requirements include flexibility of ward routines so that oral care can follow the individual's own established routines as to when, where and how they practise mouth care. It can be disorientating to introduce a system that changes these patterns or denies the opportunity for self-care[12]. With older established patterns, routines will be even more difficult to change. If the objective is to promote self-care, the first step must be the provision of facilities that will allow individuals to retain or re-establish, as much as possible, their previous routines for mouth care and even improve upon them. Although orientated to the ward setting, this checklist can be easily applied to the home and other community care environments as part of community assessment.

7.11 The requirements when assistance is needed

If the oral assessment indicates that some help will be needed with oral care in either the short or long term, a care plan should record the requirements and interventions. As oral health status will change in response to systemic factors, so the type and degree of assistance will change. The manager should be satisfied that care plans are appropriate and reviewed.

For example, a client who has suffered a cerebro-vascular accident may pass through several stages of oral dependency. Initially, he or she may be semiconscious and be fed intravenously or parenterally. At this stage, oral needs will consist of a safe receptacle for dentures (if worn); these should be labelled and stored wet in a similarly labelled container. The mouth will require appropriate oral care and frequent moistening for comfort. If dentate (possessing natural teeth), then tooth brushing and sugar free lubrication is advised.

As recovery continues and the patient returns to an oral diet, the presence of any facial paralysis or weakness will require extra attention to oral hygiene on the affected side as food is likely to accumulate. Loss of use of the dominant hand means that the patient may need help with mouth and denture care. It may be difficult to retain and control dentures due to loss of neuro-muscular control. The temporary use of denture fixative can be helpful until such time as assessment by a dentist can be organised. Adaptations to toothbrushes and denture brushes may also be needed, and assistance with tooth brushing may be necessary.

Any residual loss of function may require permanent modification of dentures and oral hygiene equipment for cleaning teeth or dentures. It is also possible that, due to unmet oral needs, the nurse will identify other long-standing problems or pathology which merit referral to the dental team. In the community setting this may entail nurses themselves facilitating referral and subsequent treatment.

7.12 Summary

In this chapter, the central roles of managers in health and social care settings have been addressed. Although much of the practical work involves others, the manager, whether in nursing or social care, is the lynchpin around whom good nursing and care practices revolve, and who has responsibility for ensuring that all members of the team have the knowledge and skill to promote and sustain the oral health care needs of their patients or clients. Nurses and health care workers are keen to improve the quality of oral care for their patients and clients as evidenced by the wealth of papers in the nursing press. Later sections dealing with specific client groups or conditions will provide the basis for the specialised training component and assist managers to comply with national guidance[1-3]. The climate is ripe for change.

References

1. DoH. Better Care, Higher Standards. A charter for long term care. 2001.

2. Department of Health. (2001). The essence of care.
    www.doh.gov.uk/essenceofcare/index/htm

3. Welsh Assembly Government. Fundamentals of Care: Guidance for Health and Social Care Staff. 2003.

4. House of Commons, Health Committee. Access to NHS Dentistry: First Report. London: The Stationary Office, 2001

5. Department of Health. NHS Dentistry: Options for Change. London: DoH, 2002.

6. Oliver CH, Nunn JH. The accessibility of dental treatment to adults with physical disabilities in northeast England. *Spec Care Dent* 1996 **16**: 204-209.

7. Edwards DM, Marry AJ. Disability Part 2: Access to dental services for disabled people. A questionnaire survey of dental practices in Merseyside. *Br Dent J* 2002 **193**: 253-255.

8. Frenkel H. Behind the screens: care staff observations on delivery of oral health care in nursing homes. *Gerodontology* 1999 **16**: 75-80.

9. Fiske J, Griffiths J, Jamieson R *et al*. Guidelines for oral health care for long-stay patients and residents. *Gerodontology* 2000 **17**: 55-64.

10. Longhurst R. A cross-sectional study of the oral health care instruction given to nurses during their basic training. *Br Dent J* 1998 **184**: 453-457.

11. White R. Nurse assessment of oral health: a review of practice and education. *Br J Nurs* 2000 **9**: 260-266.

12. Longhurst R. An evaluation of the oral care given to patients when staying in hospital. *Primary Dent Care* 1999 **6**: 112-115.

13. Adams R. Qualified nurses lack adequate knowledge related to oral health resulting in inadequate oral care of patients on medical wards. *J Adv Nursing* 1996 **24**: 552-600.

14. Roberts J. Developing an oral assessment and intervention tool for older people: 2. *Br J Nursing* 2000 **9**: 2033-2040.

15. Bowsher J, Boyle S, Griffiths J. A clinical effectiveness systematic review of oral care. *Nursing Standard* 1999 **13**: 31.

16. Collard M, Hunter L. Oral care protocols for children receiving treatment for cancer. *J Disabil Oral Health* 2001 **2**: 15-17.

17. Paulsson G, Soderfeldt B, Fridlund B *et al*. Recall of an oral health education programme by nursing personnel in special housing facilities for the elderly. *Gerodontology* 2001 **18**: 7-14.

18. Locker D. The burden of oral disorders in populations of older adults. *Community Dent Health* 1992 **9**: 109-124.

19. McGrath C, Bedi R. A study of the impact of oral health on the quality of life of older people in the UK - findings from a national survey. *Gerodontology* 1998 **15**: 93-98.

20. Roberts J. Developing an oral assessment and intervention tool for older people: 1. *Br J Nursing* 2000 **9**: 1124-1127.

21. Miller M, Kearney N. Oral care for patients with cancer: a review of the literature. *Cancer Nursing* 2000 **24**: 241-254.

22. Rawlins CA, Trueman IW. Effective mouth care for seriously ill patients. *Prof Nurs* 2001 **16**: 1025-1028.

23. Milligan S, McGill M, Sweeney MP *et al.* Oral care for people with advanced cancer: an evidence based protocol. *Int J Pall Nurs* 2001 **7**: 418-427.

24. Lee L, White V, Ball J *et al.* An audit of oral care practice and staff knowledge in hospital palliative care. *Int J Pall Nurs* 2001 **7**: 395-400.

25. Honnor A, Law A. Mouth care in cancer nursing: using an audit to change practice. *Br J Nurs* 2002 **11**: 1087-1096.

26. Barber S, Jerreat M, Jagger DC *et al.* Denture care of patients in hospital. *J Disabil Oral Health* 2002 **3**: 68-71.

27. McNally L, Gosney MA, Doherty U *et al.* The orodental status of a group of elderly in-patients: a preliminary assessment. *Gerodontology* 1999 **16**: 81-84.

28. Wilkin K. A critical analysis of the philosophy, knowledge and theory underpinning mouthcare practice for the intensive care unit patient. *Intensiv Crit Care Nurs* 2002 **18**: 181-188.

29. Travers AF, Corrado OJ, Basker RM. Geriatricians' knowledge of dental problems in older people. *Age Ageing* 1997 **26(Suppl 3)**: 33.

30. Boyle S. Holistic Oral Care in Project 2000. Oral Health Education Research Group Newsletter. 1994.

31. Charteris P, Kinsella T. The Oral Care Link Nurse: a facilitator and educator for maintaining oral health for patients at the Royal Hospital for Neuro-disability. *Spec Care Dent* 2001 **21**: 68-71.

32. Curzio J, McCowan M. Evidence based practice. Getting research into practice: developing oral hygiene standards. *Br J Nurs* 2000 **9**: 434-438.

33. Royal College of Surgeons Faculty of Dental Surgery and British Society for Disability and Oral Health. 2001. Clinical guidelines and integrated care pathways for the oral health care of people with learning disabilities. http://www.rcseng.ac.uk or http://www.bsdh.org.uk

Chapter 8

Oral effects of medication

8.1 Introduction

The principles of good pharmacotherapy involve balancing the benefits of medication against the potential risks and side-effects. Age, body weight, liver and kidney disease affect toxicity and the rate at which drugs are absorbed and excreted. The problems of compliance and the possibility of abuse must be considered. Tissues which exhibit rapid cell growth and cell turnover are more likely to be affected by the side-effects of medication. Red and white blood cells and the soft tissues of the mouth fall into this category.

The mouth is permanently populated by micro-organisms: bacteria, fungi and viruses. In a healthy person with good oral hygiene and normal salivary flow, a fairly constant balance is achieved between different micro-organisms with no evidence of oral infection. However, an upset in the balance of micro-organisms caused by poor oral hygiene, illness or medication may lead to oral infection and other distressing symptoms. The importance of saliva and its bacteriostatic and bactericidal properties is summarised in Chapter 1.

Drugs may also have a direct effect upon oral tissues and more importantly on the developing foetus, if taken during pregnancy. This chapter summarises the more important side-effects of medication on the mouth and is of relevance for anyone caring for someone on medication.

8.2 Sugar in medicines

An area of particular concern to the dental profession is the use of sugars to make drug preparations more palatable and acceptable. Liquid medicines are particularly suitable for children and anyone who has difficulty swallowing medication in tablet form. Because of the importance of extrinsic sugars in the process of dental caries, persistent and long-standing use of sugar based liquid medication is of particular concern in children with chronic illness, and any sector of the population who are dentate. Chronically sick children who suffer, or need to be protected from frequent infections are more at risk. Children with chronic illness taking long term oral medicines have significantly more dental caries of their primary anterior teeth than their siblings[1]. The prescription of sugar based medicines for the increasing number of dentate older people is also a matter of concern, and of even greater concern if they are also taking medication which causes dry mouth (xerostomia)[2].

The increase of prescribed medicine intake and of self-medication in developed countries exposes a growing number of children to medication caries, which can be considered a public health problem[3]. Drug companies have been responding to the demand for 'sugar-free' medicines. Despite the fact that the British National Formulary specifically indicates medicines that are sugar free, liquid preparations containing sugars are the most commonly prescribed by doctors and the most commonly sold over the counter by pharmacists[4]. Of 67 different liquid oral medication preparations which were used long-term, 39% were sugar-based, 33% were sugar free, and the rest 'variable'; either sugar based or sugar free depending upon how specifically they were prescribed[5].

In a study of doctors, pharmacists and health visitors, the frequency of sugar intakes as an important cause of dental caries was not well understood[6]. Continued education for health professionals is recommended to show the importance of the frequency of sugar intakes and to change prescribing practice to encourage sugar free substitutes[3,5]. Mackie[4] in an editorial in the *British Medical Journal* highlights a legislative problem; if a prescription for a generic medicine does not specify SF (sugar free) on the prescription, then a drug containing sugar will be dispensed even if both the pharmacist and the parent would prefer a sugar free preparation. So the onus is on the prescriber to specify an appropriate preparation. It is important to bear in mind that some sugar free preparations contain sugar substitutes e.g. aspartame, which might be a problem to certain patient groups. Whenever possible, the dental profession encourages the prescription of medication that is sugar free or artificially sweetened when appropriate.

Products listed in the *British National Formulary*[7] and the *Dental Practitioners' Formulary*[8] which are marked 'sugar free' do not contain glucose, fructose or sucrose. Preparations that contain hydrogenated glucose syrup, mannitol, sorbitol or xylitol are also marked 'sugar free' since there is evidence that they are not cariogenic. Any dentate patient who is prescribed medicines containing cariogenic sugars should be advised of the risk, the need for appropriate dental hygiene measures to prevent caries and the benefits of appropriate fluoride preparations (Chapter 2). It would seem obvious that giving liquid medication through a straw may reduce the potential for contact with the teeth.

More recently, the prolonged administration of glyceryl trinitrate preparations for the treatment of ischaemic heart disease have been associated with localised dental caries in the area where the tablet is retained[9]. Glyceryl trinitrate tablets contain lactulose. As the tablet dissolves slowly in the mouth, the active ingredient is released along with a relatively large amount of lactose. Although lactose in milk is considered to have a low cariogenic potential (Chapter 2), it seems that pure lactose in this form may be more cariogenic by causing a more rapid fall in the pH of saliva. Susceptible individuals who regularly use this form of glyceryl trinitrate preparation should be targeted for preventive dental advice.

Food supplements are increasingly being prescribed to ensure an adequate nutritional intake. The Formulary lists a wide range of preparations in Appendix 7 as borderline substances. Many of these preparations have a high carbohydrate content and flavouring. In order to encourage intake, cartons may be sipped at frequent intervals throughout the day. It is therefore important to check the contents for cariogenic sugars and ensure appropriate preventive measures are advised or instituted. Mackie[4] highlights this as detrimental to the dental health of children taking nutritional food supplements e.g. for young patients who are intolerant of lactose or protein. But food supplements are also a risk factor for dental caries in dentate persons of all ages, in particular older people.

8.3 Contact reactions

Toxic reactions may occur as a result of direct or prolonged contact between medication and delicate oral soft tissues. If drugs are allowed to pool in the mouth or are retained in contact with oral tissues, an inflammatory reaction may occur. Ulceration of the floor of the mouth may be caused by medicine or tablets that have not been swallowed. In older people whose oral soft tissues may be thin and atrophic, the reaction may be severe. By observing whether medication has been swallowed, it may be possible to prevent this potential complication.

Chemical burns occur due to prolonged contact of drugs with oral soft tissues. An aspirin tablet placed in direct contact with a crowned tooth for pain relief produced the chemical burn illustrated in *Figure 8.1*. Compliance with the use of medication as advised on the package is advised to avoid serious and painful reactions.

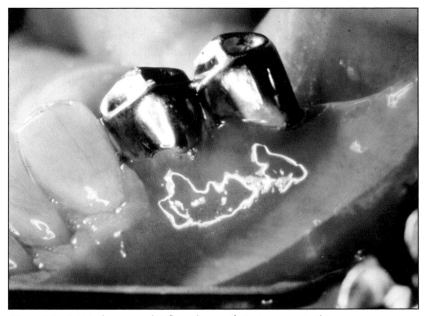

Figure 8.1 Aspirin burn: a red inflamed area of gingivae next to the crowned teeth caused by placing an aspirin tablet there for local pain relief

8.4 Drugs in pregnancy

It is well accepted that medication during pregnancy should be avoided, particularly during the first trimester, unless it is prescription medication. In the case of drugs which have been demonstrated to affect foetal development during the first trimester (teratogens), congenital malformation may affect the teeth and jaws. The degree of abnormality depends upon the dose and stage of foetal development at which the drug is taken. Perhaps the most common example of this is thalidomide. Aspirin has been associated with Reye's syndrome and is contra-indicated for children under 12 years and during breast-feeding. In the illustrated example of Reye's syndrome, there was abnormal facial development with a very high arched palate that retained plaque and debris *Figure 8.2*.

Certain drugs should be avoided during the period of tooth development. Tetracycline and its derivatives cause discolouration in the developing tooth structure and occasionally cause dental hypoplasia. Discoloured teeth may have an overall blue tinge (*Figure 1.1*). This is not damaging to teeth but may be cosmetically unacceptable. Tetracycline is no longer prescribed during pregnancy, to breast feeding women or children under 12 years of age.

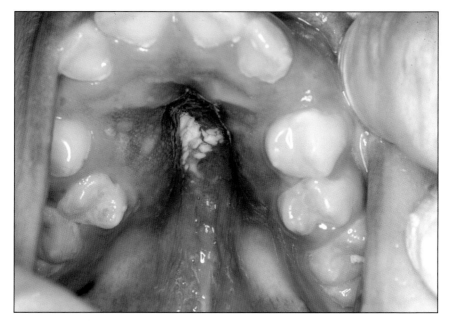

Figure 8.2 Reye's syndrome: abnormal facial development is accompanied by a very high arched palate, which can retain plaque and debris

8.5 Oral side-effects

Although the oral side-effects of drugs are relatively uncommon, it is worth noting some of the more common preparations that may be prescribed for conditions covered in Section III. In some cases, oral infections and ulceration are secondary to drug induced blood disorders. Dry mouth (xerostomia) is an uncomfortable and potentially harmful oral symptom which is usually caused by a reduction in salivary flow. Many drugs and drug classes have been linked to xerostomia. The xerostomic effect increases when many drugs are taken concurrently[10]. Drugs which reduce salivary secretions have the potential to increase the risk of dental caries, periodontal disease, oral infections and other lesions. Xerostomia has a negative impact on oral health status and quality of life, and is an important problem in older adults already compromised by chronic medical conditions. A comprehensive list of over 30 groups of xerostomic drugs categorised according to their function is provided in *Table 8.1*[10] but not all drugs which fall into these categories cause xerostomia.

Table 8.1 Xerostomic medication categorised according to function

AIDS Related Complex Therapeutic Agents	Erectile Dysfunction
Alzheimer's Disease Management	Gastric Acid Secretion Inhibitors
Analgesics	Gastrointestinal Agents
Anaphylaxis Emergency Kit	Hormone Inhibitors
Anorectic Agents (Appetite Suppressants)	Hypocalcaemia Management
Anti-arrhythmic Medications	Migraine Preparations
Anti-asthma Agents	Multiple Sclerosis Management
Anticholinergics and Antispasmodics	Muscle Relaxants
Antiemetic drugs	Nausea Medications
Anti-convulsant Medication	Opioid Antagonists
Benzodiazepine Antagonists	Osteoporosis Medication
Bronchodilators	Parkinson's Disease Medication
Cold and Cough Preparations	Peripheral Vasodilators
Coronary Vasodilators	Pruritis Medication
Dermatological Preparations	Psychotropic Medication
Diagnostic Aids	Smoking Cessation Aids
Diarrhoea Medication	Sympathomimetic Combinations
Dietary Supplements (synthetic)	Vasodepressors
Digestive Enzymes	

Based on Sreebny and Schwartz [10]

Frequency and severity of side-effects are variable and affected by the individual's general state of health, and interactions with other drugs and treatments. Some side-effects are summarised in *Table 8.2* although the list is by no means comprehensive. A detailed list of oral side-effects that may follow drug treatment can be found in Scully and Cawson[11]. Other side effects such as facial pain, erythema multiforme (Stevens Johnson Syndrome), angio-oedema, pigmentation of the oral tissues, lichenoid, lupoid and pemphigoid-loke reactions, salivary gland swelling and pain, hypersalivation, disturbed taste, red saliva, cervical lymph node enlargement and trigeminal paraesthesia are also listed. As new drugs are being developed and new side-effects reported, it is essential to check for side-effects in the current issue of the *British National Formulary.*

Table 8.2 Possible oral side-effects of medication

Side effect	Drug
Xerostomia (dry mouth)	Amphetamines Antihistamines Anti-hypertensives Anti-Parkinsonian drugs Appetite suppressants Atropine and its derivatives Baclofen Benzhexol Bronchodilators Clonidine Decongestants Ganglion-blocking agents L-dopa Lithium Monoamine oxidase inhibitors Phenothiazines Propantheline Tricyclic antidepressants
Oral infections eg Candidosis	Broad spectrum antibiotics Corticosteroids Cytotoxics Immunosuppressives Drugs which cause dry mouth
Oral ulceration	Allopurinol Cocaine Cytotoxics Gold Indomethacin Isoprenaline Penicillamine Phenylbutazone Potassium Chloride
Gingival hyperplasia (swelling)	Contraceptive pill Cyclosporin (*Figure 8.3*) Diltiazem Nifedipine Phenobarbitone Phenytoin (*Figure 11.2*) Primidone

Blistered areas	Busulphan
	Captopril
	Carbamazepine
	Clonidine
	Frusemide
	Penicillamine
	Phenylbutazone
Involuntary facial movements	Butyrophenes
	Carbamazepine
	Levodopa
	Methyldopa
	Metoclopramide
	Phenothiazines
	Tetrabenazine
	Tricyclic antidepressants
Superficial staining of teeth	Chlorhexidine
	Iron
Developmental tooth discolouration	Fluoride
	Tetracycline (*Figure 1.1*)
Dental caries	Sugar based medication
	Glyceryl trinitrate

The authors have encountered confusion amongst some health professionals; the assumption has been that medication needs to be taken orally in order to give rise to oral side-effects. It is important to note that these are systemic side-effects that may occur when medication is given orally, intramuscularly, intravenously, or parenterally.

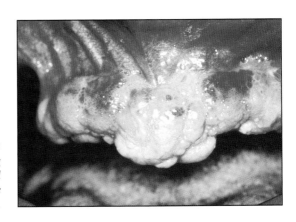

*Figure 8.3
Hyperplastia (swelling and enlargement) and inflammation in a denture wearer taking cyclosporin.*

8.6 Summary

A comprehensive account of the oral side effects of medication is beyond the scope of this book. Interactions between drugs are even more complex, and with the increasing number of new drugs that come onto the market each year, this section would become rapidly out of date. However, it is important for health professionals to be aware of the potential for oral side-effects, particularly sugar in medicines and xerostomia (dry mouth), and their implications for oral health.

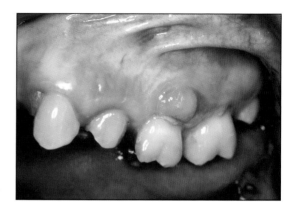

Figure 8.4
Swelling of the gingivae, a
side effect of Nifedipine

We suggest that the reader always refers to the most recent issue of the *British National Formulary* (BNF) published twice a year, to access current information on possible side-effects. Suspected adverse drug reactions should be reported to the Medical Control Agency using the yellow reporting forms or by contacting the listed Freefone Service, details of which are provided within the BNF. It is only through diligent reporting of any adverse reactions that new side-effects can be recorded. Side effects and drug interactions can also be checked by visiting the BNF website: http://www.bnf.org

References

1. Maguire A, Rugg-Gunn AJ, Butler TJ. Dental health of children taking antimicrobial and non-antimicrobial liquid oral medication long-term. *Caries Res* 1996 **30**: 16-21.

2. Field EA, Fear S, Higham SM *et al*. Age and medication are significant risk factors for xerostomia in an English population attending general dental practice. *Gerodontology* 2001 **18**: 21-24.

3. Bigeard L. The role of medication and sugars in pediatric dental patients. *Dent Clin North Am* 2000 **44**: 443-456.

4. Mackie IC. Editorial: Children's dental health and medicines that contain sugar. Doctors must take the lead by prescribing sugar free medicines whenever possible. *Br Med J* 1995 **311**: 141-142.

5. Maguire A, Rugg-Gunn AJ. Prevalence of long-term use of liquid oral medicines by children in the northern region, England. *Community Dent Health* 1994 **11**: 91-96.

6. Bentley E, Mackie I, Fuller SS. The rationale, organisation and evaluation of a campaign to increase the use of sugar-free paediatric medicines. *Community Dent Health* 1997 **14**: 36-40.

7. British National Formulary 2003. British Medical Association and Royal Pharmaceutical Society of Great Britain.

8. Dental Practitioner's Formulary 2003. British Dental Association, British Medical Association and Royal Pharmaceutical Society of Great Britain.

9. Walton AG, Rutland RFK. Glyceryl trinitrate preparation (Suscard Buccal) causes caries and changes to the denture base material. *Br Dent J* 1998 **185**: 288-289.

10. Sreebny LM, Schwartz SS. A reference guide to drugs and dry mouth – 2nd edition. *Gerodontology* 1997 **14**: 33-47.

11. Scully C, Cawson RA. Medical Problems in Dentistry. London: Butterworth-Heinemann Ltd 1998.

Chapter 9

Aids to oral self-care, rehabilitation and independence

9.1 Introduction

This chapter describes some of the equipment, therapeutic and preventive aids available to promote oral health. Advice is given on aids and adaptations to support oral self-care and to support carers in carrying out this aspect of personal care for people who are dependent or need assistance with oral hygiene. Individual oral hygiene advice lies within the remit of the dental hygienist, but this chapter will be of particular interest to a wider audience, for example occupational therapists, as it also covers aids to oral hygiene and mouthpieces for independence.

9.2 Environmental factors

Environmental factors covered in Chapter 7 fall within the remit of several disciplines and are discussed in Section 3 in relation to current legislation. Advice on design of the physical environment and equipment to facilitate independence can be obtained from the Disabled Living Foundation[1] (*Figure 9.1*).

9.3 Detection of plaque

Before considering the diverse range of products that are advertised to promote gingival health, it is helpful to visibly identify areas where plaque has accumulated. Plaque is normally invisible except in the neglected

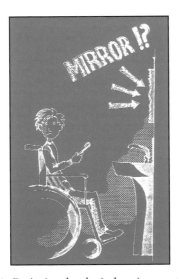

Figure 9.1 Designing the physical environment is crucial

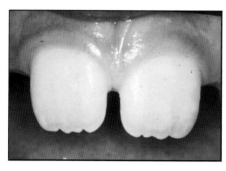

Figure 9.2a Teeth have just been brushed and appear clean and free of plaque

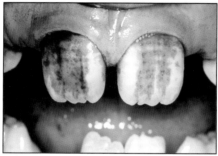

Figure 9.2b Disclosing agents reveal the invisible deposits of plaque

mouth; disclosing materials dye plaque, identifying areas that have been missed. Demonstrating plaque is useful for training and monitoring tooth brushing skills and enables the client or carer to identify areas requiring extra attention (*Figure 9.2*). Disclosing agents can be delivered as tablets for chewing or in solution. Solutions that are painted or swabbed onto the teeth may be more useful for the client or carer to use; they can be applied with cotton buds or a swab. Products which contain food dyes may be unsuitable for people with food allergies.

9.4 Toothbrushes

It is universally accepted in the dental literature that the most effective tool for mouth care i.e. removing plaque, is a toothbrush[2]. In evaluating tools currently in use for mouth care, there is general agreement that toothbrushes are superior to traditional nursing methods of care that utilise foam sticks, swabs, swabbing or topical swabs and forceps[3-5]. Despite evidence and recommendations for changes in nursing practice, in the authors' experience, toothbrushes are not universally available or used in hospital, particularly in Intensive Care Units. A child's toothbrush is more comfortable, easier to manipulate and less traumatic if correctly used. Yet when toothbrushes are issued in hospital, they tend to be of a standard size with cost being the prime factor in brand selection. Different types of toothbrush are described below.

Manual toothbrushes

Research suggests that there is no one superior design of manual toothbrush and that the user is by far the most significant variable in efficient toothbrushing[6]. Toothbrushes come in all shapes and sizes with wide-ranging claims by the manufacturers. A toothbrush should be able to remove plaque from all tooth surfaces without damaging hard or soft tissues, and fit properly into the hand. The most suitable is generally a medium or small headed brush with medium to soft nylon filaments, with the proviso that it is replaced as soon as the filaments start to splay at the tips (*Figure 9.3*). Variations in the shank, handle and angle of the head provide a wide choice for the self-caring person. Flexibility in the handle can provide greater efficiency in reducing trauma during tooth brushing. Children require a smaller head than adults. The handle of some brands can be modified by immersion in hot water, a useful feature when the angle of head to handle needs to be modified. Toothbrushes must be regarded as personal use items to prevent transmission of infection.

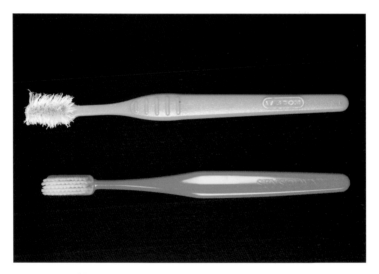

Figure 9.3 Old and new toothbrushes

A double-headed toothbrush that permits simultaneous brushing of palatal or lingual and buccal surfaces has been shown to be effective as the bristles are angulated to contact the gingival margins at the correct angle[7] (*Figure 9.4*). The handle can also be adjusted by immersion in hot water. This is useful for people who find tooth brushing tiring and for care-givers when access is difficult as both outer and inner surfaces are brushed simultaneously. A conventional toothbrush is still required for occlusal surfaces.

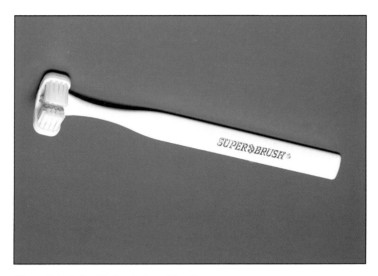

Figure 9.4 A double-headed toothbrush

Electric toothbrushes

There is a wide range of models, both rechargeable and battery operated. They are heavier than conventional toothbrushes with a wider handle and small replacement head. Brush head movement varies in different models. However the universal principle is that the brush is held in contact with each site for a specific period. All surfaces should be cleaned systematically without applying excess pressure. Powered toothbrushes with a rotary action achieve a modest reduction in plaque and gingivitis compared to manual tooth brushing if the manufacturer's instructions are followed[8,9].

Electric toothbrushes (ETBs) are considered useful for people who have lost the cognitive or manual skills, or the co-ordination to manipulate a conventional toothbrush and render the mouth plaque-free. Their efficiency depends on use but they may be no less efficient than good manual tooth brushing. If used for too short a period, they give a false sense of oral cleanliness; this is particularly true of battery operated models that lose their charge and therefore efficiency over a period of time.

A wide handle is advantageous to improve grip but the extra weight may be a disadvantage. ETBs may well have gimmick value in encouraging compliance and seem to be well tolerated by children and adults who are dependent for oral care. However, investment in what may be an expensive purchase for people who are likely to be on a low income should follow advice from the dental hygienist to ensure that the most suitable model is purchased and that it will be used correctly. Practical instruction will be required. Individual assessment of the effectiveness of plaque control with a battery operated toothbrush will provide some guidance on whether it is

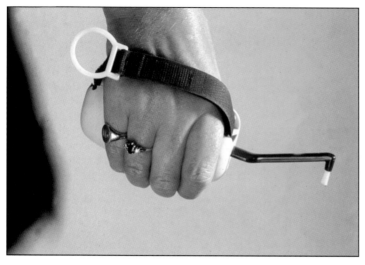

Figure 9.5 A single-tufted toothbrush

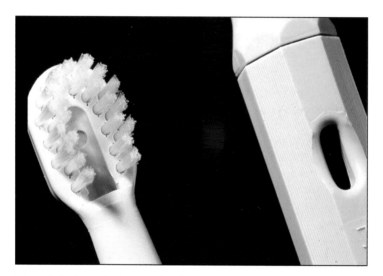

Figure 9.6 An aspirating toothbrush

a suitable for the individual and therefore an indication as to whether it may be worth investing in a more expensive re-chargeable model.

Single-tufted toothbrushes

A variety of brush heads are designed for reaching difficult areas e.g. for removing plaque from spaces between teeth, around crowns or bridges and mal-positioned teeth, and around fixed orthodontic appliances. They

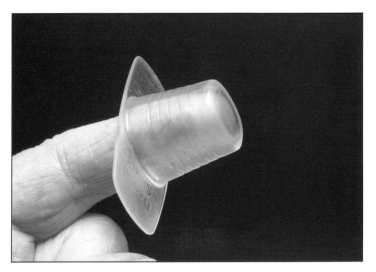

Figure 9.7 The Bedi Finger Prop, an example of a mouthprop

are designed to reach areas that standard brushes do not reach and should be used with a circular action (*Figure 9.5*).

Aspirating toothbrush

An aspirating toothbrush is useful for the dependent or dysphagic person in a nursing setting where there is access to aspiration (*Figure 9.6*). Maintaining oral health is difficult when there is risk of aspiration. Care must be taken to protect the airway. Tooth brushing stimulates salivary flow and causes frothing therefore integral aspiration has obvious benefits. It is also useful when vision is restricted and to ensure that toothpaste is not retained in the mouth. An ordinary toothbrush can be modified for use with an aspirator. The central bristles are removed and a fine Ryle's tube strapped to the handle and tied firmly to the head. However, it is not as efficient as commercially designed products.

Mouthprop

A mouthprop or bite-support made of plastic worn on the index finger of the carer's non-brushing hand can be placed between the jaws as a means of helping to keep the mouth open (*Figure 9.7*). A mouthprop is also a personal use item.

9.5 Interdental cleaning aids

Tooth brushing does not remove plaque from interdental areas or beneath

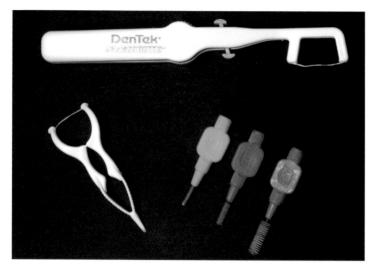

Figure 9.8 Interdental cleaning aids

gingival margins. These areas are more susceptible to decay and periodontal disease. Dental floss and tapes, and interdental brushes are designed to achieve this (*Figure 9.8*). However the nursing press makes little reference to interdental cleaning procedures in oral care.

Dental floss and flossing tapes

There are a variety of brands of dental floss and tapes designed to remove interproximal plaque. Dental floss is a fine cord, sometimes waxed and/or flavoured, sold on a reel with an integral dispenser. Waxed floss is less likely to catch or tear on rough or defective tooth surfaces, while unwaxed floss separates into several strands, providing more friction and, being finer, passes between the teeth more easily. It is claimed that elasticated floss-tape is easier to use, provides greater friction and is less likely to catch on fillings. Some brands are impregnated with Fluoride. Others brands have a stiff end to thread around and beneath bridges and fixed appliances. If used incorrectly, floss can damage the gingival tissues and over time may saw into the tooth structure. It therefore requires skill and manual dexterity to be used correctly by the self-caring individual yet few people floss correctly on a daily basis.

Flossing is difficult if not impossible for people with manual impairment. Self threaded floss holders for single use may help overcome some of the difficulties (*Figure 9.8*). The handle may need to be enlarged to ensure adequate grip and have more potential for people with restricted manual skills. They are also useful for people who are dependent for oral hygiene.

Interdental brushes

These are small fine tapered bristle brushes that clean between teeth (*Figure 9.8*). They can be hand held or mounted on a handle. They are easy use and useful for the self-caring and dependent. Again, the handle or grip may need to be modified.

9.6 Oral irrigation devices

Oral irrigation devices are designed to flush out food and debris, and reduce the concentration of bacterial plaque. Plastic syringes with a curved nozzle are less likely to cause trauma. A range of powered commercial devices exist with either a water reservoir or water-driven by attachment to a water supply. Some models have the facility to deliver antibacterial agents. They have greater cleansing efficiency and claim to stimulate gingival tissue.

These devices are useful for cleaning around fixed orthodontic appliances, wire fixation and other fixed appliances. Dependent people may benefit from their use provided that the airway is not compromised. They should not however be used on patients who are at risk of bacteraemia.

9.7 Other oral hygiene aids

These include gauze strips and pipe cleaners for cleaning wider gaps between teeth, woodsticks and toothpicks, rubber and plastic tipped devices. If used incorrectly, they may cause trauma. Their use is recommended only under the guidance of a hygienist.

Mouth packs containing foam sticks which are expensive and ineffective are no substitute for gentle tooth brushing. As the awareness of oral health increases, so new oral hygiene products appear on the market. Professional advice should be sought before purchasing new and relatively expensive aids to oral hygiene.

9.8 Toothpaste

For the dental profession, the main purpose of toothpaste is as a means of delivering topical fluoride and other therapeutic substances to the teeth and soft tissues, and as a motivator to plaque removal. The potential cosmetic and cleansing sensation may be of greater importance to the user.

The preventive importance of fluoride in toothpaste is discussed in Chapters 1-3. It is difficult for the lay person to assess the manufacturers' claims for plaque inhibition, control of calculus (tartar) and desensitisation in the ever-increasing range of new products. Fluoride containing toothpastes that contribute to enamel remineralisation are still the most widely recommended by the dental profession and the most beneficial for dental health[10]. New products are being researched for their effectiveness in reducing dentine hypersensitivity[11]. Flavoured toothpastes, provided they contain fluoride, are favoured to encourage children to brush their teeth. Whichever is used, it is important to remove toothpaste residue after brushing because it has a drying effect on soft tissues. However excessive rinsing may reduce the benefit of fluoridated toothpaste. Professional advice should be sought to confirm manufacturers' claims for new products.

9.9 Fluorides

The availability of adequate fluoride confers significant resistance to dental caries. It is now considered that the topical action of fluoride on enamel is more important than the systemic effect. Dietary fluoride supplements are covered in Chapters 2 and 3 (*Table 2.3*). Fluoride supplements are only recommended for systemic use from the age of 6 months during the period of the developing dentition provided that the natural fluoride content of the drinking water is significantly less than one part per million[12].

Self-applied topical fluorides are available as a rinse, a gel for tray application and a brush-on gel. Supervision may be necessary to ensure that fluoride rinse is retained in the mouth for the required time and then expectorated. Use must comply with manufacturers' instructions. Professional advice on the most suitable concentration and method is advised.

Sodium Fluoride, available as a 2% solution diluted for daily or weekly rinsing, also available ready diluted to 0.05% for weekly use is fairly well tolerated. It is suggested that stannous fluoride is more effective in caries reduction than sodium fluoride but it has an astringent taste, may cause gingival irritation, and is more likely to stain teeth. Stannous fluoride which is also available as a 0.4% gel for brushing can be substituted for people who cannot rinse. Neutral pH fluoride preparations of 0.5-1% are more easily tolerated by patients who have received radiotherapy affecting the mouth. Stannous fluoride gel (0.4%) applied by brushing is recommended for children under the age of 6 during cancer therapy[13] (Chapter 16).

Individual assessment is essential in selecting the most suitable topical fluoride regime if rinsing with fluoride is painful or if there are problems with compliance. Topical fluorides are particularly beneficial for children and adults at risk of dental caries therefore it is important to ensure a suitable regime is based on individual assessment and professional advice.

9.10 Mouthwashes and other preparations

Mouthwashes have a mechanical cleansing action to facilitate removal of debris and provide a subjective impression of oral freshness. Products which claim to have antibacterial or antiseptic properties, and specific oral benefits should not be toxic to oral tissues. Commercially available products sometimes contain alcohol which in the compromised patient may be toxic to oral tissues and exacerbate the condition. Agents recommended in the Dental Practitioner's Formulary are summarised[12].

Chlorhexidine gluconate

Chlorhexidine gluconate is a chemical anti-plaque agent available as mouthwash, gel and spray. A number of trials have demonstrated its long-term plaque and gingivitis reducing properties[14]. Although it has the disadvantage of staining teeth, this is reversible and easily removed professionally. Mucosal irritation is reported as a very rare side-effect, however, its demonstrated effectiveness against plaque far outweighs this. The mouthwash is available in two strengths (0.12% and 0.2%) and two flavours (normal and mint). All traces of toothpaste must be removed by rinsing before using chlorhexidine to maximise the effect in controlling bacterial plaque.

Chlorhexidine gluconate is recommended as an aid to mechanical cleansing in the initial oral hygiene phase of treatment. Recommendations for use when mechanical oral hygiene is difficult are summarised in *Table 9.1*.

Table 9.1 Recommendations for use of chlorhexidine gluconate

- **Pre and post oral surgery and periodontal treatment**
- **Fixation of the jaws**
- **Fixed orthodontic appliances**
- **People whose oral health is affected by impairment, disability or treatment**
- **Medically compromised and systemic disease affecting oral tissues**

Mouthrinses are unsuitable if swallowing is impaired. Chlorhexidine gluconate (1%) can be administered by brushing or professionally applied as a gel in splints. Chlorhexidine spray (0.2%) may be more appropriate for plaque control in people who are unable to cooperate with tooth brushing or rinsing and for areas requiring localised treatment provided there is no risk of aspiration.

Hexetidine

Hexetidine (0.1%) is marketed as a mouthwash and gargle but there is no convincing evidence that gargles are effective. It is reported to be similar in action in controlling plaque but compared with chlorhexidine, there has been very little research on this agent.

Cetylpyridium chloride

This is also marketed as a mouthwash and gargle containing 0.05% cetylpyridium chloride. It has a moderate anti-plaque effect against gram-positive bacteria. It can be used undiluted or diluted with an equal volume of water but is not as effective as chlorhexidine.

Oxygenating agents

These include hydrogen peroxide and sodium perborate. The BNF suggests their usefulness in treating acute ulcerative gingivitis (Vincent's infection or trench mouth) since the organisms involved are anaerobic. They have a mechanical cleansing effect due to frothing when in contact with oral debris. This mucosolvent property may be useful in breaking down thick and viscous saliva. Oxygenating agents are not recommended for long-term use.

Hydrogen peroxide 3% (10 volume) diluted as a mouthwash has an unpleasant taste and is modestly antiseptic. It should be used with caution since it may cause chemical burns if incorrectly diluted. Patients using hydrogen peroxide have reported dry mouth and discomfort[15]. It is not suitable for patients with mucositis whose oral mucosa is at risk of providing entry for systemic infection since it breaks down normal tissue. It is therefore not recommended for oral care in patients receiving radiotherapy, chemotherapy or bone marrow transplant.

Sodium perborate has similar properties to hydrogen peroxide, may be caustic if inadequately diluted, and there is a risk of borate toxicity due to absorption. It is contraindicated for children under 5 years and in persons suffering from renal insufficiency. It should not be used for longer than 7 days.

Sodium bicarbonate

Sodium bicarbonate has mucosolvent properties and an unpleasant taste.

It is not listed in the Dental Practitioner's Formulary as an oral therapeutic agent although it is frequently cited in nursing literature[4]. There is little evidence to confirm its usefulness as a cleansing agent. It should be used with caution as it can cause chemical burns if incorrectly diluted[16].

Povidone iodine

There is little information on 1% povidone iodine. Although listed as a gargle or mouthwash for the treatment of oral infections, it appears to have no anti-plaque activity at this dilution. Reported side-effects include mucosal irritation and hypersensitivity reactions. It should not be used for longer than 14 days because a significant amount of iodine is absorbed which can interfere with thyroid-function tests.

Thymol

Anti-bacterial activity is reported when thymol and its derivatives are used in mouthwashes at relatively high concentrations. Thymol glycerin is reported to be initially refreshing but although glycerin acts as a lubricant, its astringent effect is a contra-indication in people with xerostomia (dry mouth). Thymol preparations do not appear to offer any advantage over mouthwashes that have been demonstrated to be effective anti-bacterial agents at lower concentrations.

Sodium chloride

Isotonic saline is effective and well tolerated as a mechanical cleansing agent. A warm saline solution is recommended as a cheap mouthwash to be commenced the day following dental extractions. Sodium chloride mouthwash Co BP contains 1% sodium chloride and 1.5% sodium bicarbonate with flavouring and chloroform water; although this may be palatable, there is little evidence to suggest that it has any advantage over normal saline.

Benzydamine hydrochloride

This is reported to be effective for the relief of oral ulceration. It is available as a rinse or spray; occasional numbness and stinging are reported side-effects.

Other preparations

Lemon and glycerine swabs continue to be used in the nursing setting. Their usefulness is questionable[4]. Glycerine although lubricating is astringent, and lemon stimulates salivary secretion. Overuse may lead to exhaustion of the salivary glands and increase xerostomia. The low pH increases the risk of dental caries. Other common oral preparations may contain alcohol. They have no demonstrable benefits over known anti-plaque agents and are contraindicated in patients with a history of alcohol misuse. There is increasing interest in tea tree oil (melaleuca alternifolia) as an oral therapeutic agent in maintaining oral hygiene but as yet, research into its possible efficacy in oral health care products is still in its infancy. In the absence of professional advice, tap water is a cheap and effective lubricant, while chlorhexidine gluconate is the most effective chemical anti-plaque agent.

9.11 Saliva substitutes

Water, ice chips and atomised water sprays are simple and provide relief for dry mouth. Proprietary saliva substitutes are necessary for chronic xerostomia, particularly radiation stomatitis. Local and systemic treatments are available. Artificial saliva can provide useful relief of dry mouth. A properly balanced artificial saliva should be of neutral pH and contain electrolytes (including fluoride) to correspond approximately to the composition of saliva. Most are available as a spray but the mouth should be swabbed rather than sprayed in patients who are at risk of aspiration. Pilocarpine is listed as systemic treatment for dry mouth and dry eyes in Sjögren's syndrome and xerostomia following irradiation for head and neck cancers. Products containing fluoride are more suitable for patients who are dentate (have natural teeth). The dental profession is best placed to manage the prescribing of saliva substitutes as part of the overall management of the patient, but the Dental Practitioner's List is restricted to the prescription of Artificial Saliva DPF[12].

Artificial Saliva DPF: This corresponds to the formula of Luborant but should be prescribed generically.

Luborant: The main ingredient of luborant is sodium carboxy-methylcellulose; it also contains fluoride. It is recommended for any condition giving rise to a dry mouth but the fluoride content is of no particular benefit to patients who are edentulous (no natural teeth).

Glandosane: Glandosane is delivered by aerosol. It does not contain fluoride. It also has a high pH and is therefore only suitable for the edentulous.

Saliva orthana: This contains gastric mucin and fluoride. The mucin is porcine in origin and may be unacceptable to certain ethnic groups who do not consume pork, and people who are vegetarians. It is also available as a lozenge.

Oralbalance: This product has recently been added to the DPF. It is a saliva replacement gel and may be more suitable for patients with dysphagia. It does not contain fluoride.

Other products such as Salivace and Saliveze are delivered by spray and do not contain fluoride. Salivix pastilles do not contain fluoride but are sugar free.

9.12 Adaptations

Disability and impaired dexterity may lead to deterioration in self-care. Inability to grip, inflexible joints, restricted and un-coordinated movements may restrict oral care using conventional oral hygiene equipment. A simple adaptation may be all that is required to enable the individual to maintain their own oral care. Liaison between occupational therapist and hygienist may be necessary to ensure appropriately adapted tools. An illustrated guide to aids for oral hygiene can be found on the Mun-H-Center website[17].

Toothbrushing aids

Enlarged handles improve grip. Adaptations can be constructed from cheap and readily available materials (*Figure 9.9 and 9.10*). Epoxy resin, thermoplastic materials and silicone dental impression material can be used to adapt toothbrush handles in cases of manual deformity such as rheumatoid arthritis (*Figure 9.11*)[18]. More expensive proprietary aids are available to assist with oral hygiene (*Figures 9.12 and 9.13*).

Straps help prevent a toothbrush being dropped (Figure 9.5). Long handled holders extend the reach for individuals with inflexible or limited

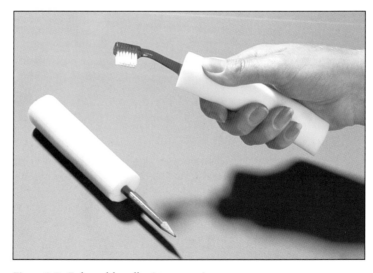

Figure 9.9 Enlarged handles improve grip

arm movements; a simple device can be constructed by lengthening the handle with a wooden splint. Occupational therapists will advise and stock a wide range of adaptations for specific problems, including splints and arm supports.

A wall mounted toothbrush holder individually constructed may benefit people with quadriplegia to maintain some control over personal care. It should not be relied on to provide effective oral hygiene without individual assessment and support from a hygienist.

Denture cleaning aids

Loss of use of the dominant hand can be frustrating for denture wearers as denture hygiene care requires two hands. Denture brushes with rubber suction cusps that adhere to the sink help to overcome this problem. A standard nailbrush can be adapted by the addition of suction cups and brushes can also be adapted to enlarge the handle (*Figure 9.14*). Proprietary products are also available and with a variety of brush heads to clean dentures (*Figure 9.15*).

Other aids

Pump-operated toothpaste dispensers, self-pasting toothbrushes and tube squeezers may overcome some problems encountered in dispensing toothpaste. A safety pin through the cap of the tube facilitates grip to remove it. Beakers with lids, lips or handles and straws may assist with rinsing and the use of mouthwashes or fluorides. The Pat Saunders drinking straw has a non-returnable valve for difficulties with sucking. It requires just a little imagination to design a simple aid or adaptation to overcome many day-to-day problems with oral hygiene. Disabled Living Centres located throughout the UK provide a useful source of advice for aids that facilitate self-care[19].

9.13 Mouth appliances for independence

People with quadriplegia or severe upper limb impairment may benefit from mouth-held devices that enable them to communicate or use environmental controls and computer systems, paint, operate lathes, operate an electric wheelchair and all manner of technical equipment to help maintain independence[20]. Mouthpieces are individually designed and involve the occupational therapist at initial and final assessment to ensure that the aid functions appropriately. Suitable end-pieces may be required for the individual's needs (*Figures 9.16 - 9.17*).

Mouthpieces generally consist of a splint which fits over the teeth to which

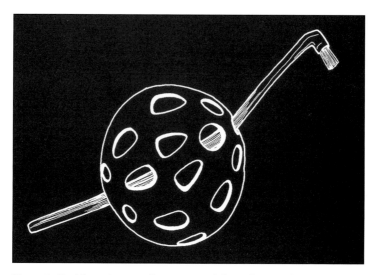

Figure 9.10 Adaptations can be constructed from cheap and readily available materials

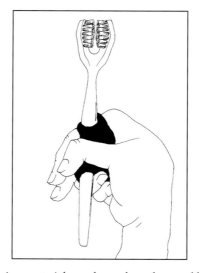

Figure 9.11 Various materials can be used to adapt toothbrush handles

various devices are attached. A healthy dentition is an advantage in designing a stable and successful mouth-controlled appliance. Oral health needs to be regularly monitored to ensure that mouth-held appliances do not damage oral tissues. Rehabilitation and independence can be significantly improved by involving the dental team.

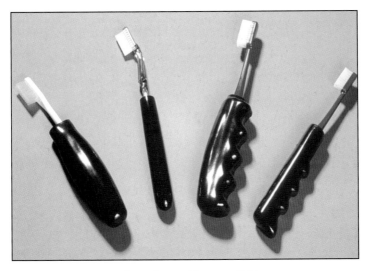

Figure 9.12 A variety of proprietary aids are available

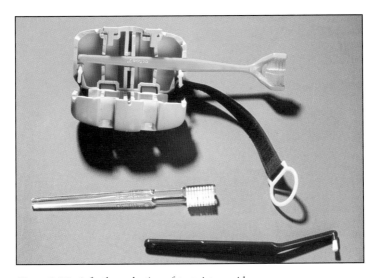

Figure 9.13 A further selection of proprietary aids

9.14 Summary

This chapter summarises information on various oral hygiene aids and therapeutic products. The self-caring individual who has regular dental check-ups should have easy access to individual oral hygiene advice from the dental team. For people with specific oral health care needs, regular oral and

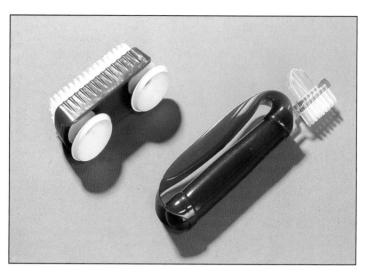

Figure 9.14 The addition of suction cups and brushes can also be adapted to enlarge the handle

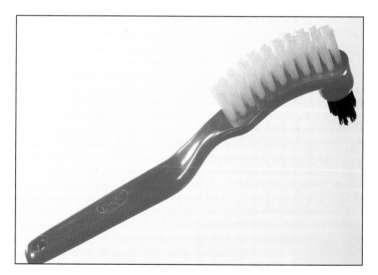

Figure 9.15 Proprietary products are also available and with a variety of brush heads to clean dentures

dental assessment will identify those areas of need that can be addressed. A home visit should be requested by people who are housebound or have an impairment that restricts their access to dental care. The dental hygienist and occupational therapist, who together provide domiciliary care and advice under the National Health Service in the UK, can monitor the use and effectiveness of aids following written referral by a dentist.

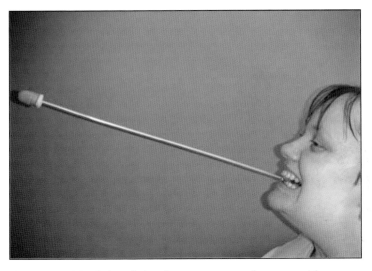

Figure 9.16 Mouthpiece designed as a page turner for person with quadriplegia; the tip can be adapted for different functions

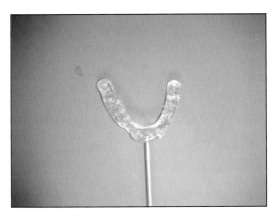

Figure 9.17 Close up of mouthpiece

References

1. Disabled Living Foundation. www.dlf.org.uk

2. Addy M, Slayne M, Wade W. The formation and action of plaque: an overview. *J Appl Bacteriol* 1992 **73**: 269-278.

3. Pearson LS, Hutton JL. A controlled trial to compare the ability of foam swabs and toothbrushes to remove dental plaque. *J Advanced Nursing* 2002 **39**: 480-489.

4. Bowsher J, Boyle S, Griffiths J. Oral care: a clinical effectiveness-based systematic review of oral care. *Nursing Standard* 1999 **13**: 31.

5. Pearson LS. A comparison of the ability of foam swabs and toothbrushes to remove dental plaque: implications for nursing practice. *J Advanced Nursing* 1996 **23**: 62-69.

6. Claydon N, Addy M, Scratcher C *et al*. Comparative professional plaque removal study using 8 branded toothbrushes. *J Clin Periodontol* 2002 **29**: 310-316.

7. Holgate W. A clinical trial to evaluate plaque removal with a double-headed toothbrush. *Br Dent J* 1991 **171**: 236-238.

8. Heanue M, Deacon SA, Deery C *et al*. Manual versus powered toothbrushing for oral health. Cochrane Database Syst Rev 2003; 1: CD002281.

9. Williams K, Walters PA, Bartizek RD *et al*. The reduction of gingivitis using battery-powered toothbrushes over a one-month period. *J Clin Dent* 2002 **13**: 207-210.

10. Clarkson JJ, McLoughlin J. Role of fluoride in oral health promotion. *Int Dent J* 2000 **50**: 119-128.

11. Sowinski J, Ayad F, Petrone M *et al*. Comparative investigations of the desensitising efficacy of a new dentifrice. *J Clin Periodontol* 2001 **28**: 1032-1036.

12. Dental Practitioners Formulary 2003. British Dental Association, British Medical Association and Royal Pharmaceutical Society of Great Britain.

13. British Society for Disability and Oral Health. Guidelines for the oral management of oncology patients requiring radiotherapy, chemotherapy and bone marrow transplantation. *J Disabil Oral Health* 2001 **2**: 3-14.

14. Santos A. Evidence-based control of plaque and gingivitis. *J Clin Periodontol* 2003 **30 Suppl 5**: 13-16.

15. Madeya M L. Oral Complications From Cancer Therapy: Part 2 - Nursing Implications for Assessment and Treatment. *Oncology Nursing Forum* 1996 **23**: 808-819.

16. Kite K, Pearson L. A rationale for mouth care: the integration of theory with practice. *Intensive Critical Care Nursing* 1995 **11**: 71-76.

17. Mun-H-Center. www.mun-h-center.com

18. Dickinson C, Millwood J. Toothbrush handle adaptation using silicone impression putty. *Dent Update* 1999 **26**: 288-298.

19. Disabled Living Centre Factsheets. http://factsheets.disabledliving.org.uk

20. Warren K. Mouthstick prostheses and other gadgets. *Dent Update* 1990 Dec: 428-430.

Section 3: At risk groups: people with specific oral health needs

This section provides information on the specific oral and dental problems of people who fall into a higher risk category for oral and dental disease, and dental treatment. It is relevant to all healthcare professionals and anyone involved in direct care and support, and concerned with prevention and health promotion.

There are numerous risk factors for oral health associated with impairment, illness, disease and treatment. Section 3 focuses on the specific needs of people in this category. Chapter 10 discusses the evolution of terminology and the requirements of the Disability Discrimination Act. Chapter 11 covers conditions that present at birth or in childhood. Subsequent chapters focus on illness and impairment in adults and medical aspects that influence oral health such as systemic, infectious and malignant disease, and mental health problems. Section 3 ends by discussing practical aspects of oral care for people who are dependent, dysphagic or seriously ill. It is impossible to classify all the causes of impairment from a social perspective so a system approach will be taken to the commonest conditions. There will inevitably be some overlap between chapters and greater focus on medical aspects of care. The essence of quality care lies in accurate assessment of the individual, and it may be necessary to dip into several chapters to find all the relevant information.

Chapter 10

Impairment, disability, handicap and specific needs

10

10.1 Introduction

There are certain individuals and groups who by virtue of illness, disease and/or treatment, impairment, disability, life-style or cultural practices are at greater risk of poor oral health. The management of dental care poses other health risks and in addition they experience barriers to the access and receipt of dental care[1].

It is estimated that there are about 500 million disabled people world wide; the majority are in the developing world[2]. The percentage of the population who have some form of disability in wealthier countries is higher as a result of improvements in neonatal medicine, advances in medical intervention, better health and social care provision and greater life expectancy. The most recent UK Census estimates that there are almost 9.5 million people in England and Wales with some form of disability[3]. This is significantly higher than previous estimates of the number of disabled people in the UK. Of these 18.2% said they had a long-term illness, a health problem or disability that limits their daily activities and opportunities for employment.

Disabled people have experienced, and continue to experience, considerable discrimination based on society's attitudes to disability (impairment or disability was and still is viewed as the cause of the disadvantage or limitations experienced by an individual). They experienced restrictions in terms of where they lived, generally confined to large institutions, in access to education, and the choices available to them in adult life. However the disability movement worldwide has challenged the concept of disability as a medical problem requiring treatment and stressed the concept of disability as a problem of exclusion from ordinary life. In the latter half of the twentieth century, the political pressure created by the disability movement generated major changes leading to increased access to mainstream education, the closure of large institutions in favour of living in the community, the right to form relationships and to participate equally in society in terms of employment, leisure and all other facets of life. This is just the first step in recognising the equality rights of disabled people. In many countries this has lead to new anti-discrimination legislation; in the UK, the Disability Discrimination Act (1995) makes discrimination on the basis of disability unlawful[4]. Despite some of these advances, the struggle to establish equal rights for disabled people will continue.

10.2 Terminology

There will be on-going discussion about the terminology associated with the labelling of different groups within society and the discrimination they experience. To understand the importance and relevance of this and to try and ensure that terminology within this text is consistent and acceptable, it is necessary to clearly define changes in terminology. In the time after this book is published, there may be new terms that are accepted as politically correct to the client group they describe. The reader should be alert to changes in terminology that are acceptable to people who experience discrimination on the grounds of gender, sexuality, race, disability or religion.

10.3 World Health Organisation (WHO, 1980)

The World Health Organisation's International Classification of Impairments, Disabilities and Handicaps gives the following definitions:

- Impairment – any loss or abnormality of physiological or anatomical structure or function
- Disability – any restriction or lack (resulting from an impairment) of ability to perform an activity in a manner or within the range considered normal for a human being
- Handicap – the disadvantage for a given an individual, resulting from an impairment or a disability, which limits or prevents the fulfilment of a role that is normal (depending on age, sex, social and cultural factors) for that individual[5].

These definitions focus on the individual or medical model of disability and concentrate on the negative aspects of what an individual cannot do rather than on the individual's functional abilities. The medical model defines and categorises disabled people by their impairment and tends to view the individual as the victim or problem, requiring rehabilitation or treatment to conform with a concept of 'normality'.

10.4 Disability Discrimination Act (1995)

In the UK Disability Discrimination Act (1995) (DDA), disability is defined functionally as:

"...a physical, sensory or mental impairment, that has an adverse effect on the individual's ability to carry out normal day-to-day activities, that the adverse effect is substantial and long-term, has lasted for 12 months or is likely to last for 12 months or a life-time"[4].

The DDA definition of disability is based on an assessment of the individual's current and potential functional capabilities. It is no longer acceptable to use impairment/ disability and disability/handicap interchangeably. The term 'handicap' is now seen as having pejorative connotations.

10.5 World Health Organisation (WHO, 2001)

The ICIDH classification was criticised by disabled people and professionals who recognised that the role of the environment was inadequately recognised in the WHO concept of disability. The WHO subsequently revised its classification to remove the negative association with handicap and to focus on participation and limitations of activity associated with impairment:

- Impairment – the functional limitation within the individual caused by physical, mental or sensory impairment
- Disability – the loss or limitation of opportunities to take part in the normal life of the community on an equal level with others due to physical and social barriers[6].

The WHO definitions provide a tool for international comparison and a framework for describing human functioning on a continuum that recognises functioning from both an individual and environmental perspective. The individual's functioning and disability is based on a dynamic reaction between health, environmental and personal factors.

The WHO goes on to provide key definitions:

- Body functions are the physiological functions of body systems (including psychological functions)
- Body structures are anatomical parts of the body such as limbs, organs and their components
- Impairments are problems in body function and structure such as significant deviation or loss
- Activity is the execution of a task by an individual
- Participation is involvement in life situations
- Participation restrictions are problems an individual may experience in life situations
- Environmental factors make up the physical, social and attitudinal environment in which people live and conduct their lives[6].

This view of disability places far greater stress upon the effect of the environment in limiting the individual's activity. It does not deny the existence of impairments that may affect people's daily lives but it shifts the emphasis onto the real barriers that affect equal participation.

10.6 Disabled people's definition of disability

Disabled people have their own definition of disability based on the 1981 Year of Disabled People:

> "Disability is the disadvantage or restriction of activity caused by a social organisation, which takes little or no account of people who have impairments, and thus excludes them from taking part in the mainstream of social activities."

Disability is therefore defined as a particular form of discrimination that leads to oppression. Barriers prevent people with impairments from being able to participate in every day activities. Environmental barriers are easier to identify and overcome; attitudinal and institutional barriers are the most difficult to identify and the hardest to remove.

10.7 Language

There has also been considerable discussion about the stigmatising and discriminatory language used to label individuals and groups. It may be stating the obvious to say that words such as a *'cripple'*, *'spastic'*, *'mongol'* or *'lunatic'* are no longer acceptable. Describing a disabled person as *'brave'* or *'tragic'*, or as *'suffering'* from a condition is also unacceptable as it defines disabled people as victims of their individual 'condition' rather than circumstance. Language and terminology are culturally sensitive. In the UK, 'learning disability' has for some time been accepted as the term to describe people with an intellectual impairment, replacing the term 'mental handicap'. However 'learning difficulty' is the term preferred by members of People First, an empowering organisation that represents this group. *Table 10.1* describes terminology that is currently acceptable to disabled people. Language which infantilises is also unacceptable. Terminology is constantly changing and it is essential that health professionals are alert to changes in terminology and review their use of language to ensure that it is neither offensive nor discriminatory.

Table 10.1 Terms that disabled people in the UK find most acceptable[7]

Disabled people / person	Acknowledgement of the way society disables people
Wheelchair user Blind people / person Deaf people / person People with Cerebral Palsy	These are accurate terms that give information about the impairment but not about the individual

Accessible: toilet
          transport
          housing
          car parking
	Facilities which are accessible to everyone, including people with impairments

Non-disabled person	Acknowledges that not everyone is discriminated against on the grounds of their impairment alone
Person with an impairment / condition	Used by medical professionals and others when talking about the individual
People with learning difficulties	Preferred term chosen by People First Organisation
Do you have any specific needs?	An open question that focuses on the individual's need not their impairment and which provides useful information
P.A. (Personal Assistance), enablers, supporters	Describes what a disabled person needs to live their life

(Alison John & Associates Ltd, 2004)

10.8 Disability Discrimination Act, 1995 - impact for dental care

The Disability Discrimination Act (1995) (DDA) is the first British statute to address the issue of disability discrimination. The legislation is aimed at ending the discrimination that disabled people experience, as, before 1995 it was lawful to discriminate on the grounds of disability. Removing the barriers to disabled people's full participation is now a legal requirement.

In 2003, in addition, the Government changed the law to ensure that people with cancer also count as a having a disability for the purposes of the Act: 'from the time at which the cancer is diagnosed as being a condition that requires substantial treatment'.

The DDA states that discrimination against disabled people is prohibited by all providers of goods and services, including providers with less than 15 employees. So the Act applies to health services and to all providers of dental services. In general terms, the DDA requires service providers to act fairly and be flexible by taking action to remove barriers that exclude disabled people. The Act also allows Government to set minimum standards so that disabled people can use public transport more easily.

The second definition of discrimination in the DDA recognises that disabled people are discriminated against as much by the barriers that an unthinking society puts up as by the attitudes of individuals. The Act requires service providers to make reasonable adjustments; the goal of the adjustment is to remove that disadvantage to create a level playing field. It refers specifically to 'less favourable treatment' which is unlawful for a reason related to disability (where it cannot be justified under the terms of the Act) even where a provider treats a person less favourably or refuses to serve them because they think this is for the disabled person's own good. From October 1st 1999, reasonable adjustments that were required included:

- Making reasonable changes to procedures and practices
- Providing reasonable auxiliary aids or services
- Providing the service by a reasonable alternative means e.g. by making a home visit.

So the Act already applies to the provision of dental care.

From October 2004, there is a requirement for service providers to take reasonable steps to remove a physical barrier, alter or avoid it, or provide the service by a *reasonable* alternative method that still enables people to make use of it. The key word within the Act is reasonable. In some situations, it may not be possible to make major physical changes but even minor changes can have a significant impact on access and communication. In broad terms, organisations with more resources will be expected to do more in terms of improving access. If a person's disability makes it unreasonable for them to attend a dental surgery to access dental services, then domiciliary dental care will become increasingly important in the legal context of the Act.

The Disability Conciliation Service (DCS) set up by the Disability Rights Commission acts as a mediator in challenges to the Act and helps avoid lengthy and expensive litigation[8]. To date, the DCS lists two cases that relate to health care; the first describes a wheelchair user who had difficulty accessing a health centre due to abuse of disabled parking bays and the second a person with vision impairment who missed appointments because correspondence was not in a reasonably accessible format. Both cases were upheld.

There are no reported challenges in relation to dental services under the DDA but the cases quoted could apply to dental services. Domiciliary dental care is not widely known about by the general public but with increasing awareness of services and rights under the DDA, it is only a matter of time before a challenge is brought under the Act.

10.9 Nature of impairment and disability

The age of onset, and the nature and degree of impairment will have an impact on an individual's ability to adjust and adapt to the current or potential limitations that they may experience. Social and environmental factors have a significant impact on abilities and limitations. Different individuals with similar impairments will face different limitations created by the social environment. Whether impairment or disability occurs in childhood, adolescence or adult life, is chronic, gradual, progressive or sudden in onset, in many individuals there is a potential impact on oral health. We are concerned about the possible impact of impairment on oral health and the social and environmental limitations that have a negative impact on oral health. Individual assessment is the foundation from which to identify the factors that act as barriers to good oral health. Subsequent chapters in this section will provide information in depth on specific oral and dental problems associated with mental, physical, medical and sensory impairment, treatments, and their impact on oral health and dental management.

10.10 Barriers to oral health

These can be broadly classified under the inter-related headings of attitude, access, and ability.

Attitude

Attitudes can be viewed from the perspective of the individual, their families, carers, and health professionals including the dental team. Attitudes underpin most health behaviour and this is also true of oral health. Attitudes to oral health and disease, the need for oral care, dietary intake of sugars, preventive regimes, regular dental attendance and the relative value placed on these factors in the context of an individual's impairment underpin this book. Other factors related to coping with impairment and disability on a daily basis may mean that oral health has a much lower priority. These factors also apply to family and professional carers. Chapters 6 and 7 have referred repeatedly to the need to change and improve the oral care practices of professional carers. It is our contention that an understanding of the impact of oral health on holistic health and quality of life may contribute towards changes in carers' attitudes and hence practice in maintaining oral health.

Many disabled people are referred for secondary dental care. Lack of confidence, training and experience may be a major factor in dentists' attitudes towards the treatment of disabled people[9,10]. Concerns about the quality of care that can be provided and the stress experienced in treating disabled patients can contribute towards negative attitudes to providing treatment[11]. Some of the reasons that are reported include:

- Lack of time
- Need for special facilities
- Inappropriate or challenging behaviour
- Inadequate remuneration for treatment which is more time consuming[12,13].

Undergraduate and post-graduate dental education is gradually addressing the perceived lack of training and experience in the specific needs of impaired and disabled people[14].

Access

Access to information, transport and services are key issues in the political debate about equal rights for disabled people and the key to independence and choice. Section 3 provides information on specific oral and dental problems. It is anticipated that making this information accessible to healthcare professionals and their patients will increase an individual's access to information relevant to his or her particular situation.

Impaired mobility leads to social isolation, which in itself is a barrier to obtaining information, and conditions people over the years to have low expectations of services. The effects of sensory impairment are also wide reaching and can lead to information deficit. However the format in which information is provided and distributed is also a barrier. Information in large print, on tape or in Braille, communication systems such as induction loops, text-phones, email and the availability of human interpreters are all covered under the part of the DDA that became law in October 1999. The technology exists but these resources are still not widely available.

In a case for anti-discrimination legislation, Barnes points out that the physical environment of mainstream housing, transport and the architectural infrastructure has been constructed without reference to the needs of disabled people[15]. Problems in finding a dentist to provide treatment under the NHS are currently being experienced by the general public. Difficulties in finding accessible dental premises are a further barrier to oral health. The main problems are caused by stairs, physical barriers within the premises and poor signage together with lack of portable dental equipment to provide a domiciliary dental service[9,13]. Without regular dental attendance, delays in obtaining preventive advice and treatment often lead to crisis management for pain relief. Section 21 of the DDA that refers to the accessibility of premises for disabled people became law on 1 October 2004.

Primary Care Trusts in England will receive funding to audit NHS dental practices in order to identify what reasonable changes can and should be made to increase accessibility for disabled people[16]. Although the DDA falls short in the eyes of many disabled people, it does place legislative pressure upon service providers. Watson argues that disabled people should not be seen as a minority group and the dental team should start examining their own practices and procedures rather than assuming that it is only and always the 'disabled' person who is the problem[2].

Ability

Ability includes the individual's physical and cognitive ability to carry out effective oral care and to seek dental services. It also includes the ability of carers, whether family, informal or professional, to provide advice and care for those who are dependent on them for personal needs or activities of daily living. In referring to dependence for oral care, we do not mean the dependence created by institutional practices. We accept the arguments of disabled people that dependence is not an intrinsic feature of impairment but is socially created by a disabling society.

In Chapter 2, it was clearly shown that effective oral care requires knowledge, skill and motivation. Many so called self-caring adults who should be able to manage their own oral care have already lost their natural teeth. If learning is restricted or impaired, or the individual lacks motivation to carry out effective oral care, an increased risk of disease is inevitable.

Caring for the mouth is just one aspect of personal care. Plaque must be removed efficiently and regularly for oral hygiene to be effective, and most people need individual advice relevant to their needs. For some people, the techniques for maintaining oral health will be more difficult to learn, and regular supervision may be required, while supervision and assistance will be essential for others. People who are severely or profoundly impaired are likely to be completely dependent with regard to maintaining oral health and therefore reliant on the knowledge and skills of their carers. They will also be dependent in terms of their dietary intake.

Without good oral hygiene, dietary control of sugars and appropriate prevention, pain is an almost inevitable consequence. In some cases, because of neglect or the individual's inability to cooperate, the ultimate outcome for pain relief will be extraction of teeth under general anaesthesia, a procedure that also has health risks. Loss of natural teeth may add an extra burden, particularly if the individual is unable or unwilling to learn the necessary skills to control and use dentures successfully. Inability to wear dentures adds a further burden that may result in social disability.

Impairment affecting upper limbs, manual control and dexterity may influence self-care in oral hygiene. Loss of use of the dominant hand will require that new skills be learnt. Poor oral hygiene and periodontal disease is found in paraplegics with diminished ability for self-care[17,18]. Aids and adaptations to compensate for impairment help to improve oral self-care (Chapter 9). Interdisciplinary assessment by an occupational therapist and dental hygienist may be necessary to identify effective aids and adaptations and assess whether personal assistance is required.

10.11 Summary

In 1988, at an international conference on oral health and disability, Justin Dart at the United States Congressional Task Force on the Rights and Empowerment of Americans with Disabilities, stated:

> "Quality dental care contributes to basic oral health and to the development of the type of self-image and social image that will be absolutely essential for the emergence of people with disabilities from an eternity of oppression"[19].

We do not have such grandiose expectations for this book, but we do hope this section in particular will provide the information necessary to promote the oral health of people with illness, impairment and disability to improve oral health, as a contribution to holistic health and health gain. In conclusion, 'Oral health and quality oral health care contribute to holistic health. It should be a right not a privilege'[20].

References

1. Griffiths J. Guidelines for Services. *In Disability and Oral Care.* pp 167-176. Ed. J Nunn. London: FDI World Dental Press Ltd., 2000.

2. Watson N. Barriers, Discrimination and Prejudice. *In Disability and Oral Care.* pp 15-20. Ed. J Nunn. London: FDI World Dental Press Ltd., 2000.

3. United Kingdom Census 2001. www.statistics.gov.uk/cenusus2001/default.asp

4. Disability Discrimination Act, 1995.

5. World Health Organisation. *International Classification of impairment, disabilities and handicaps: a manual of classification relating to the consequences of disease.* Geneva: World Health Organisation, 1980.

6. World Health Organisation. *International Classification of functioning, disability and health.* Geneva: World Health Organisation, 2001.

7. Alison John and Associates Ltd: alison.john@ntlworld.com

8. Disability Rights Commission. www.drc-gb.org

9. Oliver CH, Nunn JH. The accessibility of dental treatment to adults with physical disabilities in north east England. *Spec Care Dent* 1996 **16:** 204-209.

10. Matthews RW, Porter SR, Scully C. Measurement of confidence levels of new UK dental graduates: an approach to academic audit. *Int Dent J* 1993 **43:** 606-608.

11. Bedi R, Champion J, Horn R. Attitudes of the dental team to the provision of care for people with learning disabilities. *Spec Care Dent* 2001 **21:** 147-152.

12. Nunn J. Disability – a Context. *In Disability and Oral Care.* pp 3 – 14. Ed. J Nunn. London: FDI World Dental Press Ltd., 2000.

13. Edwards DM, Merry AJ. Disability part 2: access to dental services for disabled people – a questionnaire survey of dental practices in Merseyside. *Br Dent J* 2002 **193:** 253-255.

14. Thompson SA, Griffiths J, Hunter L *et al.* Development of an undergraduate curriculum in special care dentistry. *J Disabil Oral Health* 2001 **2:** 71-77.

15. Barnes C. Housing, transport and the built environment. *In Disabled People in Britain and Discrimination: A case for Anti-Discrimination Legislation.* London: Hurst and Co, with BCODP, 1991.

16. Department of Health. *Chief Dental Officer's Digest* 3 May 2003. www.doh.gov.uk/cdo/cdodigest3/discrim.htm

17. Lancashire P, Janzen J, Zach GA *et al.* The oral hygiene and gingival health of paraplegic inpatients – a cross-sectional study. *J Clin Periodontol* 1997 **24:** 198-200.

18. Stiefel DJ, Truelove EL, Persson RS *et al.* A comparison of oral health in spinal cord injury. 1993 **13:** 229-235.

19. Dart JW. Ensuring the rights of persons with disabilities. *Spec Care Dent* 1988 **8:** 245-248.

20. Clark CA, Vanek EP. Meeting the health care needs of people with limited access to care. *J Dent Educ* 1984 **48:** 213-216.

Chapter 11

Impairment in childhood

11.1 Introduction

This chapter examines the oral and dental problems, which may be experienced by people with a range of impairments that commenced at birth or during childhood.

Apart from a few conditions, people with this range of impairments will encounter the same oral and dental diseases as the rest of the population. There are additional factors such as access to dental care and support in carrying out activities of daily living, which can result in higher levels of tooth loss and untreated disease.

11.2 Cerebral palsy

Cerebral palsy (CP) is one of the major causes of physical impairment. It has been described as 'a disorder of movement and posture due to a defect or lesion of the immature brain'[1]. Other impairments associated with CP include visual, hearing and speech impairment, epilepsy and learning difficulties. The condition affects 1:500 children by school age in industrialised countries but the level and type of impairment depends on the areas and degree of brain damage. Cerebral palsy results in a wide spectrum of disability ranging from virtually unnoticeable physical impairment involving one limb (monoplegia) through to all four limbs (quadriplegia). Movement may also be affected in the following groups:

- Spastic; increased muscle tone contractions and difficulty with head control
- Athetoid; involuntary movements and difficulty with balance
- Ataxia; difficulties with balance and co-ordination.

Chidren with CP may have a mixture of the above groups.

Oral factors in cerebral palsy include:

- Malocclusion
- Bruxism (*Figure 11.1*)
- Attrition
- Swallowing, gag and cough reflex
- Acid regurgitation
- Feeding and dietary factors
- Jaw dislocation
- Effects of medications.

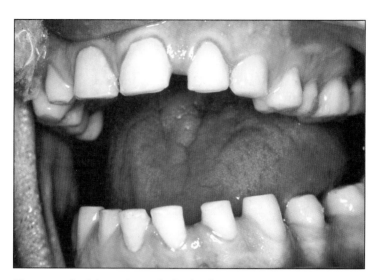

Figure 11.1 Oral factors in cerebral palsy: bruxism

Oral developmental abnormalities may affect oral health. Malocclusion, caused by irregular teeth or overcrowding, is common with delayed eruption of the teeth as a contributory cause. Factors associated with difficulties with the process of eating and digestion can result in a diet of soft and minced food. The use of dietary supplements and laxatives with very high sugar content can produce extensive levels of caries very rapidly in the absence of effective oral hygiene procedures. Without the normal oral processes of chewing and swallowing food can be retained in the mouth. The increasing use of PEG (Percutaneous Endoscopic Gastronomy) feeding has helped with improving nutritional status but the need for regular oral hygiene can be overlooked. The effects of some anticonvulsant drugs can produce gingival hyperplasia (*Figure 11.2*). Xerostomia is a side effect of some antispasmodic medications and anticholinergic drugs given to reduce drooling.

Oral and dental disease in cerebral palsy

Children with CP appear to experience higher levels of dental caries and plaque as compared to the rest of the population. Feeding problems, clearing residual food and malocclusions combined with mouth breathing appear to contribute to the higher levels of dental and oral disease. They also experience more extractions and untreated disease[2].

11.3 Learning disability

Learning disability is a collective term to describe a greater difficulty in learning than others of the same age. Another definition commonly used

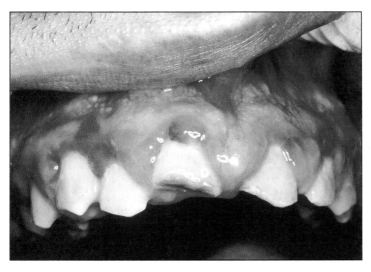

Figure 11.2   The effects of some anticonvulsant drugs can produce gingival hyperplasia (Phenytoin hyperplasia)

is: "a significant impairment of intelligence and social functioning acquired before adulthood[3]".

It can cover learning in a specific area as seen in dyslexia, dyspraxia and attention deficit and hyperactivity disorder (ADHD), or a more global learning difficulty seen in Down syndrome, autism, cerebral palsy and other congenital or genetic disorders. The process of identification of a learning disability in a child has improved over recent years. Approximately 5% have some degree of learning disability, mild, moderate or severe with the majority being males[4].

Oral and dental disease in people with learning disability

There does not appear to be much difference in the prevalence of dental caries between children with and without impairments. However children with a disability are more likely to have untreated disease and have teeth extracted more frequently. There is also a higher prevalence of dental caries in children with a mild learning disability compared to those in special schools and institutions. This is attributed to lower access to cariogenic foods and a more comprehensive approach to dental care[5]. There are many studies demonstrating a poor standard of oral hygiene and plaque control in children with learning disabilities. Again, the poorest levels are seen in those with a mild learning disability not receiving regular dental treatment.

Adults with a mild learning disability are often not in regular contact with dental services and studies of those attending day centres and institutions show higher levels of untreated decay and periodontal disease than the general population[6].

Oral health care for people with learning disabilities

The key to improving oral health for people with learning disabilities is via effective prevention and adequate access to dental services. Children and their families are in contact with a wide range of health and education professions and an integrated approach involving the dental team will ensure more comprehensive care. Clinical guidelines and integrated care pathways for the oral health care of people with learning disabilities have been published by the British Society for Disability and Oral Health and the Faculty of Dental Surgery, Royal College of Surgeons of England[7]. These provide detailed guidance for everyone involved in the care of people with learning disabilities. The guidelines focus on integrated care for:

- Pre-school children
- School age children
- Transition from adolescence to adulthood
- Adults and older people.

At each stage, evidence based guidelines are provided for:

- Prevention and promotion of oral health
- Oral assessment and care planning
- Management of specific conditions
- Training and education for parents and carers.

11.4 Down syndrome

Down syndrome is the most common genetic cause of learning disability and is caused by a chromosomal abnormality with an incidence of 1:6-800 live births. The incidence increases with maternal age, rising as high as 1:37 at 44 years. Down syndrome can be diagnosed in pregnancy with maternal and foetal blood testing. Apart from the characteristic physical appearance of a short stature and facial characteristics, there are medical and physical aspects that can affect oral health and dental management.

Some of the medical aspects of Down syndrome include:

- Congenital heart disease
- Respiratory disease

- Atlanto-axial (cervical spine) instability
- Immunodeficiency
- General anaesthetic risk
- Leukaemia
- Early onset Alzheimer's disease.

These factors can have implications for oral and dental care.

Some of the oral factors in Down syndrome include:

- Abnormal jaw relationships
- Cleft lip and palate
- Malocclusions
- Reduced masticatory ability
- Poor lip posture
- Mouth breathing
- Large tongue (hypotonic) and tongue thrusting
- High arched palate
- Abnormal shaped crowns of teeth
- Missing teeth
- Gingival hyperplasia from anticonvulsant medication.

Oral and dental disease in Down syndrome

There is an increased susceptibility to periodontal disease[8] in this group, compounded by difficulties in maintaining a good standard of oral hygiene due to anatomical factors. Lower levels of dental caries have been reported[9] which may be due to a higher pH of saliva and the small, more spaced teeth.

11.5 Autistic Spectrum Disorders (ASD)

Autism is a collective term for a range of disorders and is now more often known as Autistic Spectrum Disorder (ASD). In the UK the prevalence rate is 9:1,000 people. Although there are four times as many boys affected, girls tend to be more severely affected.

The condition is usually diagnosed by the age of three years. There are difficulties with verbal and non-verbal communication, with forming relationships and often other signs, such as repeated body movements. There are also associations with learning difficulties, epilepsy and Down syndrome. There are no obvious causes of autism aside from a possible genetic link and although there has been considerable publicity regarding a possible link with the MMR vaccine, there does not appear to be any conclusive evidence one way or another.

A consistent characteristic feature of people with ASD is that they like routine. They may also have a very short attention span and a need for continuity. An exaggerated sensitivity to smells and lights may also be present.

Asperger's syndrome is part of the Autistic Disorder Spectrum. However, language and communication skills are not as affected. People with Aspergers are likely to have good intellectual ability but may have a short attention span. Children with this syndrome can have poor co-ordination and delayed development of motor skills.

Oral and dental disease in Autistic Disorder Spectrum

There is little general difference in childhood levels of dental disease. Some children may have higher levels of caries from receiving sweets to reward behaviour. Conversely, some children may be on restricted diets due to either their own wishes or due to parents finding that sugars and food additives adversely affect their behaviour.

Short attention span and need for continuity can affect the way that dental care is provided, as extra planning is needed. People with more severe aspects of ASD may have difficulties tolerating dental care[10].

11.6 Muscular dystrophy

Although diseases affecting the musculature are relatively uncommon, muscular dystrophy (MD) is the most common in childhood. Of these, Duchenne muscular dystrophy is the most common, the most severe form and is progressive from early childhood, affecting 1:4,000 male births. Becker type, which is less disabling, progresses more slowly and mobility is less likely to be affected. There are several other rarer forms, which are classified by the groups of muscles affected. In myotonic dystrophy, which occurs mainly in adults, facial weakness, speech and swallowing difficulties may occur. Children with muscular dystrophy may also have scoliosis and learning difficulties; one form is associated with epilepsy.

Oral and dental disease in muscular dystrophy

There are no specific oral features, although malocclusions due to widening of the jaw arches may occur. This is caused by the greater pressure of the tongue in relation to the weakness of lip and cheek muscles. Delayed eruption of teeth is also sometimes seen. The 'open mouth' posture due to weakness in the facial muscles is a risk factor for oral health. The resultant dryness of the mouth and difficulties in maintaining self-care due to upper limb weakness increases the risk factors for dental caries and periodontal disease. Swallowing difficulties may complicate oral care. The respiratory and cardiac problems are a risk factor for general anaesthesia[11].

It is important to provide training and education for parents and carers as support for oral self-care is required.

11.7 Rickets and osteomalacia

Rickets is mainly caused by a deficiency of vitamin D. This can lead to a failure in bone formation. Rickets occurs in children; the disease in adults, osteomalacia, presents mainly during pregnancy and lactation. The deficiency is mainly due to a dietary deficiency of meat, oily fish and a lack of exposure to sunlight, and had largely disappeared in the UK. It is now seen more often amongst recent immigrants who have suffered malnutrition and ethnic minorities, related to cultural food and dress practices. In children the bones are weak and prone to fracture and deformity. In adults it affects the weight-bearing bones[12].

Oral and dental disease in rickets

There may be delays in the eruption of teeth, although tooth structure is rarely affected except in severe cases.

11.8 Rheumatoid arthritis and juvenile arthritis

Rheumatoid arthritis is an acutely disabling disease, which affects all ages, with females more frequently affected than males. It has a variable course, but is generally progressive with severe inflammation. Swelling with acute pain and joint deformity usually affects hands and feet and later knees, ankles, wrists and elbows. In the active phase anaemia is common.

Approximately 15% of people with rheumatoid arthritis develop Sjögren's syndrome, the symptoms of which are dry mouth and eyes.

When the temporomandibular joint is affected, mouth opening may be limited. See Chapter 12 for a more comprehensive review of rheumatoid arthritis in adults and details of oral and dental disease.

Juvenile rheumatoid arthritis is rare, but severely disabling. It affects 10:100,000 children[13]. There are a number of different types, of which Still's disease is one, in which approximately half develop severe and chronic impairments.

11.9 Osteogenesis imperfecta (brittle bone disease)

As lay terminology for this rare condition implies, brittle bone disease is a disorder in which bone is extremely fragile and prone to multiple fractures, particularly in childhood. This arises from a defect in the collagen fibres forming the infrastructure for bone formation. Although the fractures heal rapidly, permanent physical deformity may result from repeated fractures. It is usually inherited, although in 25% of cases children are born into families with no history of the disorder. There are four types of the disorder with symptoms ranging from mild to severe. The range of problems associated with the condition include:

- Early hearing loss
- Bruising
- Respiratory problems
- Dentinogenesis imperfecta (underdeveloped dentine in teeth).

Treatment of the condition involves managing the fractures and encouraging mobility by splinting or the insertion of metal rods in the long bones.

Oral and dental disease in osteogenesis imperfecta

Approximately half the people with osteogenesis imperfecta also have dentinogenesis imperfecta, often referred to as opalescent teeth. The teeth are bluish and prone to wear. Malocclusions and delayed eruption are often seen. Extensive restorative dental care is often required[14].

11.10 Spina bifida and hydrocephalus

Spina bifida and hydrocephalus may occur together or independently. Spina bifida is a congenital defect caused by incomplete development of the spinal neural tube. It is a collective term that covers three conditions of varying severity:

- Spina bifida occulta
- Spina bifida cystica menigocele
- Spina bifida cystica myelomenigocele.

Spina bifida occulta does not cause any physical or neurological abnormality. The two forms of spina bifida cystica are a major cause of paraplegia in children and usually require surgical correction. Other complications can include:

- Hydrocephalus
- Congenital hip dislocation
- Epilepsy
- Learning difficulties.

Spina bifida occulta is present in 5-10% of the population, but is usually not noticeable. Spina bifida cystica is present in approx. 1:1,000 pregnancies. There is a gender variation of 3:2 women to men and an increased incidence among some ethnic groups.

The condition appears to be caused by environmental and genetic factors. Folic acid taken during pregnancy can significantly reduce the incidence. History of a sibling with spina bifida is an increased risk as is an adult having a child with spina bifida[15].

Hydrocephalus

Hydrocephalus is caused by obstruction to the circulation of cerebrospinal fluid. It may be secondary to congenital conditions, infections, haemorrhage or tumours and can cause brain damage due to pressure or atrophy. Unless treated, hydrocephalus leads to enlargement of the skull, brain damage or death. Epilepsy, visual impairments, spasticity and learning difficulties or dementia may present as complications.

The condition is treated by the insertion of a valve to divert cerebrospinal fluid away from the area and to reduce pressure. Valves may become dislodged or blocked and require regular monitoring.

Oral and dental disease in spina bifida

There are no specific oral or dental factors associated with spina bifida except how paraplegia and complications may affect access to services. There is a high incidence of latex allergy among people with spina bifida and antibiotic cover may be required to protect potential infections of the valve[16].

11.11 Sensory impairments

The major sensory impairments are loss, or reduction of sight, hearing or both. Total deafness in childhood is rare and the commonest cause of conductive deafness is often due to chronic secretory otitis media following recurrent middle ear infections. Some groups are at higher risk including people with cleft lip and palate, and Down syndrome. Conductive deafness is often intermittent and can resolve with no treatment. Sensorineural hearing loss occurs in 1:1,000 births. It is usually present from birth and results from damage to the cochlea, auditory nerve or other abnormality. It is more profound and may be progressive. It may follow infections such as measles or meningitis and is a feature of many syndromes.

Visual abnormalities occur in 1:3,000 births. There are genetic causes for 50% of severe visual impairments. Other causes include infections, trauma and retinopathy related to premature birth. Children can also have a combination of hearing and visual impairment.

Oral and dental disease and sensory impairments

There are no specific factors in oral and dental disease associated with sensory impairments. However there may be problems accessing appropriate dental care and maintaining oral health due to difficulties with communication. This can result in higher levels of untreated dental caries and periodontal disease, and complications receiving dental care[17].

11.12 Cleft lip and palate

Cleft lip and palate is one of the commonest forms of congenital developmental disorder affecting the oral cavity. The defect can range from a small notch in the upper lip to a complete cleft affecting lips, hard and soft palate. Cleft lip and palate can occur together or separately and affect approximately one in every 700 births per year in the UK. Incidence varies within different racial groups; approximately 1 in 1000 Caucasians are affected by this condition, whereas cleft palate alone affects 1 in 2,500 people. Cleft lip is more common in males, and cleft palate is common in females.

Although most cases are of genetic origin, cleft lip and palate may occur in association with other syndromes or developmental disorders. Although the causes of the condition are not well understood, environmental factors such as drugs, infections, maternal illness, maternal smoking and alcohol use, nutritional and vitamin deficiencies are possible causative factors. Thalidomide is reported to be associated with clefts and is a known teratogen. Clefts may also be associated with other congenital conditions, notably Down syndrome, and much rarer conditions, many of which are associated with a learning disability.

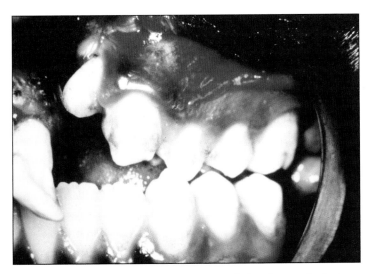

Figure 11.3 Cleft lip and palate in a young male immigrant who had not received early surgical treatment in his native land. Facial disfigurement and embarrassment while eating led to psychological problems and withdrawal. These problems started to resolve after corrective cosmetic surgery

Problems associated with cleft lip and/or palate have consequences for feeding, speech, communication and learning, as well as the psychological effects of potential facial disfigurement and social acceptance. Hearing may be affected as a result of increased susceptibility to middle ear infections leading to mild to moderate hearing loss; this can also complicate the development of speech, interfere with social development and delay learning.

The degree of involvement depends upon the severity of the cleft and structures affected. Clefts may involve just soft tissue or both hard and soft tissues, and may be unilateral or bilateral. The more complex the defect, the greater the potential for oral impairment. Facial deformities are the most obvious visible signs, while feeding difficulties may pose major problems in early childhood, particularly if the palate is affected (Chapter 18). The use of appliances designed to cover the palatal defect and assist with feeding in early childhood is controversial[18]. Obturators are necessary to close the palatal defect in adults with un-repaired clefts.

Surgical repair of cleft lip is carried out at an early age, usually around three months, while palate repairs are generally completed by about 15 months, before development of speech[18]. Complex repairs may require multiple operations at various developmental stages; these may be complicated by medical problems associated with other abnormalities. Susceptibility to upper respiratory tract infections may require frequent medication; the effect of sugar based medicines and the potential for dental caries is highlighted in Chapters 3 and 8. Missing and mal-aligned teeth lead to problems with occlusion. Orthodontic treatment to correct abnormalities may be started early but is usually carried out when the permanent dentition is fully erupted[19].

Cleft lip and palate if untreated pose a major risk of oral impairment (*Figure 11.3*). Assessment and treatment planning is usually implemented very soon after birth; the ideal multi-disciplinary team will include as core members, the surgeon, orthodontist, speech and language therapist and ENT specialists. However a comprehensive cleft lip and palate service should also include dental services, specialised counselling services and clinical genetics in the team[20]. Preventive programmes to include fluoride supplements in areas without water fluoridation, dietary advice and the development of good oral hygiene techniques are vital and should be implemented from birth. All professionals involved in the care and treatment of patients with clefts must be aware of the need and availability of lifetime preventive oral health advice. The Cleft Lip and Palate Association (CLAPA), a voluntary organisation providing advice and support for people affected by cleft lip and palate is an excellent source of information[21].

11.13 Summary

In this chapter we have described a range of early onset impairments. Many of the conditions that are present at birth or commence in childhood will, of course, have implications in adulthood due to improvements in treatment and ongoing care.

References

1. Bax MCO. *Develop Med & Child Neurol* 1964 **6:** 295-297.
2. Dos Santos Mt, Masiero D, Novo NF *et al.* Oral conditions in children with cerebral palsy. *ASDC J Dent Child* 2003 1970 **1:** 40-46.
3. Clinical guidelines and integrated care pathways for the oral health care of people with learning disabilities. 2001. P1. www.bsdh.org.uk
4. Lyon GR. *Future child* 1996 **6:** 54-76.
5. Clinical guidelines and integrated care pathways for the oral health care of people with learning disabilities. 2001 P7. www.bsdh.org.uk
6. Clinical guidelines and integrated care pathways for the oral health care of people with learning disabilities. 2001. P14. www.bsdh.org.uk
7. Clinical Clinical guidelines and integrated care pathways for the oral health

care of people with learning disabilities. 2001 P7-24. www.bsdh.org.uk

8. Lopez-Perez R, Borges-Yanez SA, Jimenez-Garcia G *et al.* Oral hygiene, gingivitis and periodontitis in persons with Down's Syndrome. *Spec Care Dent* 2002 **22:** 214-220.

9. Stephens AJ, Sapsford DJ, Curzon ME. *Br Dent J* 1993 **175:** 20-25.

10. Klein U, Nowak AJ. *Pediatr Dent* 1998 **20:** 312-317.

11. Symons AL, Townsend GC, Hughes TE. Dental characteristics of patients with Duchenne Muscular Dystrophy. *ASDC J Dent Child* 2002 **69:** 277-283.

12. Scientific Advisory Committee on Nutrition. Subgroup on Maternal Child Nutrition. Vitamin D Deficiency in Children p2-7. Dept of Health. 2003.

13. Prahalad S, Glass D. Is juvenile rheumatoid arthritis/juvenile ideopathic arthritis different from rheumatoid arthritis? *Arthritis Res* 2002 **4 (Suppl):** 303-310. www.arthritis-research.com

14. Dental care for persons with OI. www.osteo.org

15. Spina bifida, FAQ. www.neurosurgery.com

16. Hudson ME. Dental surgery in paediatric patients with spina bifida and latex allergy. *AORN Journal* 2001 July.

17. Champion J, Holt R. Dental care for children and young people who have a hearing impairment. *Br Dent J* 2000 **189:** 155-159

18. Rivkin CJ, Keith O, Crawford PJ *et al.* Dental care for the patient with a cleft lip and palate. Part 1: From birth to the mixed dentition stage. *Br Dent J* 2000 **188:** 78-83.

19. Rivkin CJ, Keith O, Crawford PJ *et al.* Dental care for the patient with a cleft lip and palate. Part 2: The mixed dentition stage through to adolescence and young adulthood. ***Br Dent J*** 2000 **188:** 131-134.

20. Shaw W, Williams AC, Sandy JR *et al.* Minimum standards for the management of cleft lip and palate: efforts to close the audit loop. *Ann R Coll Surg Engl* 1996 **78:** 110-114.

21. Cleft Lip and Palate Association (CLAPA) www.clapa.com

Chapter 12

Impairment in adults – mucoskeletal disorders

12.1 Introduction

This chapter covers the more common mucoskeletal conditions that cause impairment and disability in adults. It focuses on conditions that usually present after childhood and medical factors that influence oral health, dental management, dental attendance and dependence for oral care including diet and oral hygiene. Despite the desire to retain a focus on the social model of disability, it is inevitable that all chapters in this section will have a medical focus that overlaps with other chapters.

Mucoskeletal is a term that describes conditions affecting bones, joints, ligaments and connective tissues. It includes osteoporosis, and the large number of arthritic and related conditions (over 200) that affect more than 7 million adults in the UK[1]. Oral side effects of medication used for treatment are summarised in *Table 12.1*.

12.2 Osteoporosis

Osteoporosis is caused by a reduction in bone mass and density leading to increased risk of fracture, back pain, weight loss and curvature of the spine. An estimated 3 million people in the UK are affected: 1 in 12 men and 1 in 3 women over the age of 50 will have osteoporosis[2]. High risk groups are older people who have suffered a low impact fracture, people receiving treatment with cortico-steroids, women with early menopause or hysterectomy and those with a family history of hip fracture. Each year the numbers of people with osteoporosis experience over 70,000 hip fractures, 50,000 wrist fractures and 40,000 spinal fractures. It is therefore a significant cause of impairment that can affect mobility and self-care.

Osteoporosis is considered a major risk factor for periodontal disease[3]. The associated problems of ageing and the oral side-effects of cortico-steroids are important considerations (Chapter 8). However alendronic acid, a bisphosphonate treatment in post-menopausal women may cause severe oesophageal reactions such as ulceration and erosions leading to dysphagia and therefore have an impact on nutritional intake. When prescribed this drug, patients should be advised to stop taking the medication if these symptoms occur.

12.3 Arthritis

Arthritis is one of the biggest causes of disability in the UK, affecting people of all ages, and in particular older people. It is the most common cause of physical impairment. It is estimated that there are more than 7 million adults (15% of the UK population) with a long-term health problem associated with arthritis and arthritis related conditions[1]. Pain is a common and distressing symptom. Although there are many different forms, osteoarthritis and rheumatoid arthritis are the main causes of impairment.

12.4   Osteoarthritis

Osteoarthritis (OA), the commonest condition affecting synovial joints such as hips, knees and digits affects approximately 3 million people in the UK[1]. It is a source of pain and the cause of loss of movement. Osteoarthritis is not an inevitable consequence of ageing but does appear to be strongly age related. Although uncommon under the age of 45, risk factors include obesity, genetic factors, female gender, disease and previous trauma. Symptom relief is provided by analgesics and anti-inflammatory drugs, physiotherapy, and joint injections with cortico-steroids. Pain and restricted mobility may be treated by surgical joint replacement. Post-operative anticoagulation may affect dental management. There are no reported oral symptoms associated with OA although medication may have oral side-effects. The case for providing antibiotic prophylaxis following prosthetic joint replacement is weak and the risk of providing antibiotic cover may be greater than the risk of joint infection[4].

12.5   Rheumatoid arthritis

Rheumatoid arthritis (RA) is a multi-system disease that affects all ages, and females more frequently than males. Around 387,000 people in the UK have RA, roughly 0.8% of the population[1]. It is an auto-immune disease with a variable course but usually progressive with severe joint inflammation. Stiffness, swelling, acute pain, and joint deformity usually first affect hands and feet, and later knees, ankles, wrists and elbows. The temporo-mandibular joint (TMJ) may be involved with pain, tenderness over the joint, difficulty in chewing, reduced opening capacity and other TMJ symptoms. Pain in the TM joint is not common even in people with severe RA. During the active phase of RA, anaemia is common (Chapter 14).

Approximately 15% of people with RA develop Sjögren's syndrome, the symptoms of which are dry mouth and dry eyes. Dry mouth (xerostomia), its consequences and treatment are covered in several chapters. Added complications of drug side-effects and restrictions to self-care imposed by manual impairment can exacerbate painful and distressing oral symptoms. There is evidence of a significant association between rheumatoid arthritis and periodontal disease[5].

Oral ulceration may occur secondary to anaemia associated with an acute phase of RA or secondary to drug therapy. Aspirin, cortico-steroids, penicillamine, NSAIDs, gold and anti-malarial drugs are prescribed for symptom relief and a range of newer drugs is also available[6]. Methotrexate has been added to the arsenal for treatment because of its immunosuppressive and anti-inflammatory effects. A fatal drug interaction may occur if a penicillin is prescribed to a patient taking methotrexate[3]. Long-term use of medication can lead to serious oral manifestations (*Table 12.1*). An increase in steroid medication may be required to cope with potentially stressful situations such as dental treatment. Good oral hygiene, relief of dry mouth and other symptoms are essential for the prevention and alleviation of oral discomfort. Dental management can be affected by:

- TMJ involvement leading to restricted opening
- Cervical vertebrae involvement
- Steroid therapy
- Anticoagulant therapy following joint replacement
- Drug interactions
- Reduced ability for self-care.

12.6 Ankylosing spondylitis

Ankylosing spondylitis (AS) is a chronic, painful, progressive rheumatic disease, which mainly affects the spine. Inflammation occurs at the site of ligament or tendon attachment. This is followed by bone erosion and subsequently new bone develops. Movement becomes restricted due to new bone formation and fusion of the vertebrae. Other areas such as eyes, lungs, heart and bowel can be involved. Each year 200,000 people with AS consult their GP. The ratio of men to women is 5 to 1[1]. Around 90% of European Caucasians with AS possess the HLA-B27 gene compared with only 6% of the general population[1]. Infection is the most likely trigger. The onset of AS is gradual with back pain and stiffness over weeks or months. Hips, knees and ankles may also be affected and restricted chest expansion may limit respiration. Cardiac disease may develop in approximately 10% of people with AS and 10% may also develop TMJ involvement[7]. Pain relief is mainly achieved with non-steroidal anti-inflammatory drugs (NSAIDs) (*Table 12.1*). General anaesthesia may present risks because of cardiac disease, impaired respiratory function and restricted mouth opening.

12.7 Paget's disease (Osteitis deformans)

Paget's disease is a fairly common bone disorder of metabolic origin affecting approximately 750,000 to a million people in the UK, normally older people, and predominantly males[8]. It is characterised by bone enlargement and bone deformity. Unlike healthy bone, the structure is irregular and consequently weaker and prone to fracture. As the condition progresses, skull enlargement and spinal curvature may develop causing pressure on adjacent nerves resulting in muscle weakness. Severe skull enlargement creates pressure, which can result in deafness, visual disturbance, dizziness and tinnitis. In its mildest form the disease has no symptoms but in more severe cases, pain can be intense. Complications include arthritis and fractures. If facial bones are involved, the maxilla (upper jaw) is more commonly affected than the mandible (lower jaw). Fortunately, only a small proportion experience significant symptoms. Treatment is with bisphosphonates and more rarely calcitonin given by injection (*Table 12.1*).

Paget's disease poses problems for dental management. Whereas teeth are not visibly affected, radiographs may reveal resorbed roots or areas of excessive cementum deposits around the roots; dental extractions may therefore be more difficult. In the earlier stages of Paget's disease, excessive bleeding may follow dental extractions; in later stages, reduced blood supply increases the risk of post-extraction infection and the possibility of chronic suppurative osteomyelitis. Surgical extractions, prophylactic antibiotics and haemorrhage control complicate dental treatment. Dentures may need to be replaced or modified more frequently.

12.8 Gout

Gout is a metabolic disorder that causes acute, intermittent and painful attacks of arthritis in the joints of the foot, knee, ankle, hand and wrist. If untreated, attacks become more frequent, prolonged and generalised. It is the most common cause of inflammatory joint disease in men over 40 years of age. The big toe is the first joint affected in 70% of cases. Gout occurs most frequently in males between the ages of 40 and 60, particularly in those who are overweight or genetically predisposed. Diets high in protein and alcohol are associated with this condition (Chapter 17). Treatment is based on counselling for life-style changes. Acute attacks are treated with NSAIDs and colchicine. Long-term management is with allopurinol, probenecid and sulfinpyrazine. Oral side effects must be considered.

12.9 Lupus erythematosus (SLE)

Lupus erythematosus or lupus is an auto-immune disease that causes inflammatory changes which can affect joints, skin, kidneys, heart, lungs, cardiovascular systems and the central nervous system. The most common symptoms are extreme fatigue, arthritis, unexplained fever, skin rashes and kidney problems. Lupus runs in families, affects more women than men, and is more common in women of African American, Hispanic or Asian descent than in Caucasian women[1]. Although the cause is unknown, a combination of genetic, environmental and possibly hormonal factors are considered to be contributory. At present there is no cure for this immune system disorder, which is characterised by periods of relapse and remission.

Lupus is a broad term that covers several forms of this condition. Systemic lupus erythematosus (SLE) affects many systemic areas. It usually affects people between the ages of 15 and 45 years, although it can occur in childhood and in later life. Discoid lupus erythematosus refers to a skin disorder in which a red, raised rash appears on the face, scalp or elsewhere on the body. The butterfly or malar rash which presents over the cheeks and bridge of the nose is relatively uncommon. Rashes may have raised margins, which are scaly and can lead to scarring. Drug-induced lupus is caused by specific medications such as hydralazine procainamide; it generally resolves when medication is stopped. Neo-natal lupus is a rare form of lupus affecting newborn babies whose mothers have SLE or other immune disorders.

Oral problems that present in SLE include areas of erythema, erosions and white patches that are often symmetrical in pattern, and ulcers in the gingival margins. Sjögren's syndrome may also occur in association with SLE. Dental management can be influenced by anaemia, bleeding tendencies, cardiac and renal disease (Chapter 14), and the side effects of medication (Chapter 8). The possibility of infective endocarditis following invasive dental treatment must be considered if there is SLE endocarditis.

Treatment is mainly with anti-inflammatory medication (NSAID) and steroids. A new range of anti-inflammatory drugs called COX-2 inhibitors (celecoxib, rofecoxib and meloxicam) have fewer gastro-intestinal side effects but have a range of possible oral side-effects. Anti-malarials can cause lichenoid lesions or in some cases, oral pigmentation. Steroids have oral side-effects and affect dental management (*Table 12.1*).

Table 12.1 Possible oral side-effects of drugs prescribed for the treatment of muco-skeletal conditions

Medication	Possible oral side-effects
Allopurinol	Taste disturbances
Aspirin	Ulceration, bleeding Anaemia
Cortico-steroids	Oral candisosis (thrush)
Penicillamine	Ulceration Loss of taste
Gold	White patches
NSAIDs	Ulceration White patches Pharyngitis (Celecoxib) Mouth ulcers (Rofecoxib)
Antimalarials: Chloroquine Hydroxychloroquine	White patches
Iron	Discolouration of teeth or dentures
Methotrexate	Gingival hypertrophy (enlargement) Ulcerative stomatitis
Ciclosporin	Gingival hyperplasia
Sulfasalazine	Stevens-Johnson syndrome Stomatitis, parotitis
Bisphosphonates (Alendronic acid)	Oesophageal ulceration and dysphagia
Calcitonin	Unpleasant taste

12.10 Polymyositis and dermatomyositis

Polymyositis is an inflammatory muscle disease that causes varying degrees of decreased muscle power. It has a gradual onset and generally begins in the second decade of life. Muscle weakness and pain are the most common symptoms. Mobility is eventually impaired and dysphagia may become a problem. This condition may be associated with collagen, vascular, autoimmune or infectious disorders. When there are associated skin lesions, the condition is known as dermatomyositis. It affects children and adults, and females more often than males. These conditions are more severe and resistant to therapy in individuals with cardiac or pulmonary involvement. Prednisolone is the first line of treatment for both conditions. Immunosuppressants such as azathioprine and methotrexate may be helpful when prednisolone is not effective. Weakness of the pharyngeal muscles, steroids and any other associated disorders affect dental care.

12.11 Summary

This chapter summarises some of most common causes of mucoskeleteal impairment in adults, and specific oral problems, which pose an increased risk of oral disease together with possible oral side-effects of treatment. The oral side effects of long-term medication are identified. Many rarer conditions have not been covered but the same principles can be applied to oral health problems in other mucoskeletal conditions.

References

1. Arthritis Research Campaign. Arthritis: The Big Picture. 2002. www.arc.org.uk
2. National Osteoporosis Society. What is osteoporosis? – Factsheet. 2003. www.nos.org.uk
3. Greenwood M. Meecham JG. General medicine and surgery for dental practitioners. Part 8: Mucoskeletal system. *Br Dent J* 2003 **195:** 243-248.
4. Seymour RA, Whitworth JM, Martin M. Antibiotic prophylaxis for patients with joint replacement – still a dilemma for dental practitioners. *Br Dent J* 2003 **194:** 649-653.
5. Mercado FB, Marshall RI, Klestov AC *et al.* Relationship between rheumatoid arthritis and periodontitis. *J Periodontol* 2001 **72:** 779-787.
6. Treister N. Glick M. Rheumatoid arthritis: a review and suggested dental care considerations. *J Am Dent Assoc* 1999 **130:** 689-698.
7. Scully C, Cawson RA. Mucoskeletal disorders. In: *Medical Problems in Dentistry.* P310-335. Oxford: Butterworth-Heineman, 1998.
8. National Association for the Relief of Paget's Disease. Paget's disease: The facts. 2002. www.paget.org.uk

Chapter 13

Neurological and sensory impairment

13.1 Introduction

This chapter covers the commonest conditions that cause neurological and sensory impairment. Neural damage can cause both motor and sensory dysfunction, and higher function may also be affected if there is cerebral involvement. Some forms of neurological impairment such as dementia and Alzheimer's disease are covered in Chapter 17 which addresses the oral health needs of people with mental health problems. Sensory impairments are also referred to in Chapter 11.

13.2 Multiple sclerosis

Multiple sclerosis (MS) is a common and complex neurological condition that occurs as a result of degeneration of the myelin sheath and causes interruption in sensory and motor nerve transmission. MS is the most common cause of severe disability in young adults in the UK. The incidence of MS is estimated to be approximately 1.8 per 1000[1]. Women are more frequently affected than men in a ratio of 3:2[2]. Diagnosis is usually between the age of 20 and 40; it relies on two occurrences of symptoms involving different areas of the nervous system, at least 2 months apart, and each lasting for at least 24 hours; diagnosis is confirmed by neurological tests. Many factors are involved in MS, but no single cause has been identified. Environmental factors such as viral or bacterial infections, a genetic predisposition to MS, family history of MS, climatic and geographic factors are all relevant. There is growing evidence to suggest that infection may play a role[3]. There are four main types of MS:

- Benign MS
- Relapsing / remitting MS
- Secondary progressive MS
- Primary progressive MS.

MS is a condition characterised by remission and relapse. Although some symptoms are common, there are no typical symptoms that apply to all cases. Symptoms vary from a very mild manifestation in the benign form to steadily worsening symptoms without remission in primary progressive MS. Symptoms vary in severity and duration, and depend upon the areas of the central nervous system affected. They include fatigue, muscle weakness, tremors, double or blurred vision, ocular or facial pain, auditory giddiness, sensory loss, mobility impairment due to loss of balance, sensory loss, speech and swallow impairment, bowel and sexual dysfunction. Cerebral involvement may affect memory, motivation, insight, personality, touch, hearing, vision and muscle tone. Trigeminal neuralgia is commonly associated with MS with a reported prevalence of up to 32%[4]. For this reason, a dentist may be the first person to suspect a possible diagnosis of MS in younger persons[5]. Epilepsy in people with MS is three times more common than in the general population[6]. Symptoms and treatment of MS influence oral health, self-care and dental management. They include:

- Chronic pain: Paraesthesia
                      Dysaethesia
                      Hyperanaesthesia
                      Anaesthesia
                      Trigeminal neuralgia
- Spasticity and spasm
- Tremor
- Speech disorders
- Cognition and depression
- Fatigue
- Dizziness and vertigo
- Dysphagia
- Mobility impairment
- Side effects of medication.

People with MS experience the same oral and dental problems as the general population. However they may be more prone to periodontal disease and an increased risk of dental caries due to reduced ability for self-care and the oral side-effects of medication, particularly xerostomic medication[5,7,8] (*Table 13.1*). Dietary advice, preventive measures, aids to oral hygiene and support for carers are a priority in progressive and severe MS. Dental treatment should be arranged to coincide with the periods of remission and times of least fatigue. The patient with MS is the expert in their condition and should be consulted on how he or she prefers to manage their symptoms.

There has been considerable concern that exposure to mercury in dental filling materials can cause neurological disorders, and particularly MS. Although there is no scientific evidence to support this contention, it has lead to demand for removal of amalgam fillings. Patients should be reassured that even the MS Society advises that there is lack of proof that mercury is a factor in MS. It is reasonable to use appropriate alternative filling materials that do not contain amalgam when fillings need to be replaced but the routine removal of amalgam fillings should be discouraged; a new awareness campaign has been set up with this objective[9].

Table 13.1 Medication used in treatment of neurological disorders

Medication	Prescribed for	Oral side effects
Amantadine	Fatigue	Occasional dry mouth
Anticholinergics	Incontinence	Dry mouth
Antidepressants (tricyclics, MAOIs, SSRIs)	Depression	Dry mouth
Antihistamines	Dizziness and vertigo	Dry mouth
Azathioprine	Delaying progression of disability	Blood dyscrasias
Baclofen	Spasticity	Dry mouth
Benzodiazepines	Dizziness and vertigo	Dry mouth
Beta-Interferons	Delaying progression of disability	Possible blood dyscrasias
Botulinus toxins	Spasticity	Possible dry mouth, dysphagia and pooling of saliva
Cannabis	Alleviation of spasticity, spasm, tremor and bladder control	Xerostomia, 'fiery red gingivitis', white gingival patches, papilloma, candisosis, epithelial dysplasia, oral and pharyngeal carcinoma
Carbamazepine	Pain relief, trigeminal neuralgia	Blood dyscrasias Stevens-Johnson syndrome
Corticosteroids	Acute exacerbations of MS	Oral candidosis
Cyclophosphamide	Delaying progression of disability	Ulceration
Cyclosporin	Delaying progression of disability	Ulceration
Desmopressin	Nocturnal enuresis	
Diazepam	Muscle spasm	Salivation changes
Isoniazid	Tremor	Blood dyscrasias; rarely dry mouth
Methotrexate	Delaying progression of MS	Blood dyscrasias; ulcerative stomatitis

Oxcarbazine	Pain relief, trigeminal neuralgia	
Oxybutinin	Incontinence	Dry mouth
Phenytoin	Pain relief, trigeminal neuralgia, epilepsy	Gingival hyperplasia Erythema multiforme Involuntary facial movements Lupoid reactions Oral ulceration Rarely Stevens-Johnson syndrome
Pyridoxine	Countering side-effects of isoniazid	
Scopolamine	Dizziness and vertigo	Dry mouth
Sildenafil	Impotence	Not in BNF but other drugs for impotence cause dry mouth
Tizanidine	Spasticity	Dry mouth

Modified from Fiske, Griffiths & Thompson[5]. Reproduced from Dental Update by kind permission of George Warman Publications, (UK) Ltd

13.3 Myasthenia gravis

The name 'serious muscle weakness' is an accurate description of myasthenia gravis (MG), which is caused by defective neuro-transmission mechanisms. Weakness is at its worst following exercise and at the end of the day, and seriously affects the musculature of the face, neck, hands and feet. Generalised muscle weakness and fatigue affects mobility, speech, and swallow. MG is commoner in women in younger age groups and in men in later life. Congenital or inherited myasthenias are rare and present in childhood.

Typically the mandible (lower jaw) drops due to muscle weakness. Eating becomes an effort and dietary changes to facilitate mastication may result in an increased intake of soft or cariogenic food and an increase in tooth-food contact time. Oral self-care may be tiring and difficult. Dental care when necessary should be planned to coincide with periods of least fatigue. General anaesthesia should be avoided as respiration may be depressed.

With appropriate treatment, 90% of patients return to normal function. Symptom relief for MG is provided with anticholinesterases, a range of drugs that increase salivation. Atropine may be prescribed to reduce salivary secretion and counter the side-effects of high doses of anticholinesterase. Steroids also provide relief and their oral side-effects must be considered.

13.4 Motor neurone disease

Motor Neurone Disease (MND) describes a group of related conditions affecting motor neurones, the brain and spinal cord. MND is a steadily progressive disabling condition. Degeneration of motor neurons leads to weakness and wasting of muscles. Symptoms depend upon the site of affected motor neurones but there is no sensory or intellectual impairment. The physical aspects of weakness and muscle paralysis are the main factors for oral health and dental management. Weakness of head and neck muscles pose a risk to the airway, create eating and swallowing difficulties, and challenges for oral care. Adequate lubrication is essential to maintain comfort. If the airway is compromised, techniques described for dependent and dysphagic patients should be applied (Chapter 18).

13.5 Guillain-Barré syndrome

Guillain-Barré Syndrome (GBS), also called acute inflammatory demyelinating polyneuropathy and Landry's ascending paralysis, is an inflammatory disorder of the peripheral nerves. The cause is unknown but thought to be viral in origin. GBS is characterised by rapid sudden onset of weakness and often, paralysis of arms, legs, facial and respiratory musculature. It is a common cause of rapidly acquired paralysis. Although many cases are mild, extensive paralysis is possible in severe cases and artificial ventilation may be necessary. In the acute phase, bilateral facial palsy and dysphagia may occur, with variable motor and sensory loss in limbs. Some 10-30% have a range of residual disabilities[10]. Individual assessment at intervals during illness, rehabilitation and in recovery ensures that the most appropriate oral care is provided (Chapter 18).

13.6 Cerebrovascular accident

Cerbrovascular accidents (CVA), commonly called strokes are a common cause of impairment and disability, particularly in older people. Approximately 100,000 people in England and Wales experience a first stroke each year. It is estimated that a third will die in the first year, a third will make a good recovery and a third will be left with moderate to severe disabilities[11]. Stroke can affect all age groups; the majority are people over

55. Around 300,000 people in the UK are living with stroke related disabilities.

A stroke (CVA) may be caused by haemorrhage (cerebral or subarachnoid), thrombosis or embolism. Symptoms and prognosis are dependent on the cause, affected area and extent of brain damage. Hypertension and atherosclerosis are possible precursors for haemorrhagic and thrombotic CVA.

Subarachnoid haemorrhage affects any age group. In 50%, onset is characterised by a sudden and severe headache followed by rapid loss of consciousness[10]. Physical or emotional stress are contributory factors. In 10% of cases, the cause is a congenital aneurysm in the circle of Willis[10]. Bleeding into the cerebral ventricle is generally fatal. Approximately one third die from the first haemorrhage. Prognosis is poor but has been improved by surgical and radiological treatment.

Thrombosis and embolism are the main causes of an ischaemic stroke (CVA). Thrombotic strokes may be preceded by Transient Ischaemic Attacks (TIA), 'mini-strokes' caused by temporary interruption to the cerebral blood supply. Onset of cerebral thrombosis is generally gradual with ill-defined symptoms. Prognosis ranges from minimal impairment to death within a week[10]. Embolic causes of CVA are associated with atrial fibrillation and infective endocarditis, and are characterised by sudden onset associated with headache and immediate symptoms.

Symptoms of CVA include weakness, loss of balance, motor and sensory loss, paralysis, speech and swallowing difficulties, and intellectual and communication impairment. Common deficits affecting communication are dysphasia, dysarthria and dyspraxia, loss of visual field due to homonymous hemianopia, and sensory inattention which can involve more than one modality. In hemipleagia, personal care may be affected by loss of use of the dominant hand. Rehabilitation involves the development of new compensatory skills. Intellectual impairment delays and interferes with rehabilitation. Unilateral facial paralysis mainly affects the mandible; oral hygiene may deteriorate on the affected side due to loss of neuromuscular control and food pocketing. Previously functional dentures appear to lose their fit due to loss of neuromuscular control. In some cases, dentures can be modified to compensate for this[12].

Swallowing difficulties may increase tooth-food contact time and increase the risk of dental caries. Dietary adjustment to maintain nutritional status and facilitate safer swallowing may increase the risk of dental caries. Patients receiving parenteral nutrition are still at risk of oral disease; calculus appears to form more rapidly in tube-fed subjects compared with the non-tube fed, indicating a significant oral care need[13]. Palatal training devices may improve the swallow reflex (Chapter 18), although recovery and improvement may be spontaneous.

Predisposing factors such as diabetes may influence oral health. Thrombotic and embolic strokes are treated with anticoagulants, which affect management of dental care. Anticoagulant dosage may need to be adjusted before invasive dental treatment but the risk of lowering a patient's INR must be weighed against the risk of thrombosis[14]. Most patients on anticoagulant therapy can be managed without risk and without adjustment of anticoagulant dosage[15].

Interdisciplinary assessment should be carried out as early as possible to ensure that oral factors are included in the rehabilitation programme. Minor adjustments to dentures to improve stability or compensate for paralysis are relatively simple, and can make a significant contribution to well-being. An oral care programme that takes account of assessed and changing risk factors, side-effects of medication and nutritional intake should be implemented at the point of diagnosis.

13.7 Bell's palsy

Bell's palsy is the term for paralysis of facial muscles caused by inflammation in the stylomastoid canal. Paralysis may also develop following trauma, surgery or other serious conditions. Bell's palsy is generally preceded by pain in the area and fairly rapid onset paralysis. It is usually unilateral and may be associated with loss of taste. With incomplete paralysis, the prognosis for full recovery is good but is less favourable in cases of complete paralysis[10].

Permanent paralysis can cause drooling on the affected side. This may be reduced by fitting an intra-oral appliance to lift facial musculature or by modifying dentures; both methods having psychological benefits. Speech and swallow may be affected. As with any cause of paralysis of oro-facial musculature, food retained on the affected side is in increased contact time with teeth, thus increasing the risk of caries and periodontal disease. Short courses of steroid therapy are beneficial.

13.8 Trigeminal neuralgia

Trigeminal neuralgia (TN), also known as *tic douloureux* is a disorder of the fifth cranial nerve. It is characterised by intense stabbing pain across the face in areas supplied by the trigeminal nerve. Atypical TN is less common and may cause less intense, constant, dull burning or aching pain. TN is usually unilateral but sometimes experienced bilaterally. Onset is most often after the age of 50 but cases are known in children and even infants[16]. Facial stimuli can provoke an intense attack; it is considered to be one of the most painful afflictions. Drug therapy is the initial treatment and anticonvulsants such as carbamazepine and phenytoin are the first choice. Baclofen, pimozide, oxcarbazepine, sodium valproate and clonazepam are alternatives if symptoms are not controlled. Some anti-depressants offer significant pain relief. If drug therapy is not effective, neurosurgical procedures may offer relief. The oral side-effects of medication must be considered (*Table 13.2*).

Table 13.2 Drug treatment for trigeminal neuralgia

Baclofen	Disturbed taste Dry mouth
Carbamazepine	Erythema multiforme
Clonazepam	Salivation changes
Phenytoin	Gingival hyperplasia Erythema multiforme Involuntary facial movements Lupoid reactions Oral ulceration
Pimozide	Dry mouth Lupoid reactions

13.9   Huntington's disease

Huntington's disease (HD) is a hereditary disorder of the central nervous system caused by a chromosomal defect. It usually develops in adulthood in the 30-50 age group and is characterised by involuntary movements and progressive dementia. There is a 50:50 chance of inheriting the gene and subsequently developing HD. Symptoms may be present for some time; diagnosis is aided if there is a family history of HD. Later in the illness, symptoms include speech and swallow difficulties, weight loss, emotional changes, mood swings and depression. Cognitive changes may result in loss of drive, concentration, initiative and organisational skills.

Medication is directed at controlling involuntary movements, depression and mood swings. Butyrophenone, phenothiazines and anti-depressants may help; oral side-effects include dry mouth (*Table 13.3*). Feeding and eating difficulties arise from choreiform movements of the face and neck.

Loss of neuro-muscular control can make eating a frustrating experience. Dysphagia may lead to a change in the consistency of diet. The Huntington's Disease Association recommends a high calorie diet supplemented by high calorie drinks and 'lots of sugar'[17]; this increases the risk of dental caries. Recommended dietary changes and deterioration in oral hygiene skills combined with the oral side-effects of medication place the person with HD in a high risk category for oral disease. It is essential to try and maintain the dentition as loss of neuro-muscular control and uncontrolled involuntary movements give a poor prognosis for success in using dentures. Dental management is affected by the patient's ability to cooperate. Prevention of caries and periodontal disease should have a high priority (Chapter 2).

Table 13.3 Drug treatment for Huntington's disease

Butyrophenones eg Benperidol, Droperidol, Haloperidol	Involuntary facial movements Dry mouth
Phenothiazines	Dry mouth
Antidepressants	Dry mouth

13.10 Parkinson's disease

Parkinson's disease (PD) is a progressive neurological condition affecting movement. It is characterised by tremor mainly affecting hands and arms, rigidity, abnormal posture, dyskinesia (involuntary movements), bradykinesia (slowness initiating and executing movement) and akathasia (muscular rigidity). Hand tremor is characterised by pill rolling and is worse at rest. Arms are rigid, flexed and held at the side; bradykinesia leads to restricted mobility. Rigidity leads to abnormal posture and restricts activity, particularly in the activities of daily living. Lack of facial expression is reflected in a mask-like appearance. Speech and communication may be affected. Intellectual impairment occurs in 30-40% of cases after 7-10 years.

PD occurs most commonly in people over the age of 50 although young onset PD starts before the age of 40. Around 120,000 people in the UK have PD; approximately 10,000 people in the UK are diagnosed each year[18]. Idiopathic Parkinson's disease is caused by a deficiency of the neurotransmitter, dopamine. Other causes of Parkinsonian symptoms include cerebrovascular disease, head injuries, encephalitis lethargica, some toxins or drugs, particularly phenothiazine and butyrophenone neuroleptics[10,19].

Treatment is mainly with drugs. With early diagnosis, selegeline may delay progress of the disease. Other drugs used singly or in combination are listed with possible oral side effects (*Table 13.4*). Levodopa in combination with a dopa-decarboxylase inhibitor is the treatment of choice for idiopathic Parkinson's disease. Anticholinergic drugs relieve hand tremor at rest. Dopamine agonists (e.g. amantidine, bromocriptine, amantadine, lisuride, ropinirole and pramipexole) are prescribed when levodopa is ineffective. Facial dyskinesia, involuntary movements of the facial muscles such as pursing the lips and 'flycatcher tongue' are distressing side-effects of treatment. Physiotherapy and physical aids help maintain independence. Dietary intake is increasingly important to achieve optimal nutrition, address swallowing difficulties and lessen the symptoms of the disease.

Table 13.4 Possible oral side-effects of drug treatments for Parkinson's disease and Parkinsonian symptoms

Drug	Possible oral side-effects
Apomorphine Hydrochloride	Dyskinesia
Bromocriptine	Dry mouth
Cabergoline	Dry mouth
Co-beneldopa	Abnormal involuntary movements, taste changes
Co-careldopa	Abnormal involuntary movements, taste changes
Entacapone	Dry mouth
Levodopa	Abnormal involuntary movements, taste changes
Lisuride	Dry mouth
Pergolide	Dry mouth
Pramipexole	Dyskinesia
Procyclidine	Dry mouth
Ropinirole	Dyskinesia
Selegeline Hydrochloride	Dry mouth, stomatitis, sore throat (Mouth ulcers reported with Zelapar taken orally)

Oral problems associated with PD include:

- Xerostomia and root caries
- Dysphagia and drooling
- Neuromuscular control of dentures
- Maintenance of oral hygiene[20].

Frequent intakes of high calorie dietary supplements increase the risk of dental caries. Neurological symptoms affect dental management. Drooling and pooling of saliva is associated with delayed swallow and poor posture. A physiotherapy assessment may be beneficial to improve posture and reduce drooling. Side-effects of anticholinergic medication may help reduce hypersalivation. Botulinum toxin injections into the parotid salivary gland are helpful in reducing salivation but there is a risk of producing permanent dry mouth[19]. Burning mouth syndrome is also more common in PD[21]. As with all progressive neurological conditions, advice and prevention at diagnosis provide the best prognosis for maintaining oral health.

13.11 Spinal and cranial neurological disorders

In modern industrial society, trauma is one of the most common causes of spinal cord damage and brain injury, mainly road traffic accidents, domestic and industrial accidents and sports injuries. Rarely, spinal nerve damage may be due to infections, haemorrhage, transverse myelitis, tumours or following spinal surgery. Acquired brain injuries (ABI) refers to non-degenerative injury occurring since birth and caused by external force or metabolic derangement. It includes traumatic and non-traumatic causes such as stroke, tumours, infections, hypoxia, metabolic causes and toxins. The symptoms of acquired brain injuries are similar to those caused by trauma.

13.12 Spinal injuries

Unlike many other causes of impairment and disability, spinal cord injury (SCI) occurs predominantly in younger age groups. Although there are no accurate statistics, it is suggested that there are 30,000 to 40,000 people with SCI in the UK. The annual incidence is 750 to 1000. It predominantly affects males (approximately 86% of SCI affects males) and the main causes, which help to clarify male predominance, are:

- Road traffic accidents (RTA)   39%
- Domestic and industrial accidents   24%
- Sporting accidents   17%

- Non-traumatic   16%
- Self-harm and physical assault   4%[22].

The sudden onset and potential severity of impairment can understandably lead to a severe emotional reaction which influences the individual's ability to adjust to changes in life-style, choice and possible dependence for personal needs.

The site and severity of lesions governs the degree of impairment. Cervical lesions are the most serious. Paraplegia refers to spinal damage below the cervical vertebrae, resulting in paralysis of lower limbs. Tetraplegia (quadriplegia) refers to cervical injury resulting in paralysis of all limbs and trunk to varying degrees. With incomplete transection of the spinal cord, limited function and sensation may return. With lower cervical injury, arm movements may be possible, although hands may be weak, lack power and dexterity (*Table 13.5*). Postural hypotension is a complication of high level tetraplegia. Apart from functional and sensory impairment, pain, tremor, spasticity and urinary infections require medication. Antibiotics, muscle relaxants and analgesics should be checked for potential side-effects. Botox is increasingly used to treat muscle spasm and reduce trismus. Nutritional status must be maintained to prevent pressure sores.

Tetraplegia associated with high cervical lesions and intercostal paralysis may require supported respiration or tracheostomy, and a high level of dependence for activities of daily living (ADL). Cough and gag reflexes may be affected. It is important to ensure that appropriate oral care is implemented at the outset. In early rehabilitation, oral hygiene techniques may be limited to those described in Chapter 18. With lower cervical injury, adaptive equipment to support or stabilise the wrist, provide arm support and facilitate grasp may be required (Chapter 9).

SCI does not result in cognitive defects unless there is associated cranial trauma. It is generally considered to be a stable condition with life expectancy comparable to non-disabled cohorts. However there is evidence to suggest that people with SCI may feel the effects of ageing a little earlier eg. osteoporosis possibly due to lack of weight bearing, increased risk of pressure sores and deterioration of bladder function. A high proportion of people with SCI are wheelchair users. Most will be capable of full time employment but due to physical access and employers' attitudes, unemployment is high.

Poor oral hygiene and gingivitis is reported in paraplegics with diminished ability for self-care.[23,24] Dependent tetraplegics expressed problems with access to dental facilities and dry mouth as side-effects of medication.[25]

Oral self-care skills must be individually assessed; self-care must be encouraged by a team approach and the appropriate aids (Chapter 9) and support provided. The dental team may be involved in restoring fractured or decayed teeth, developing oral care plans, providing preventive advice and treatment, and in the construction of mouth appliances to promote independence (Chapter 9). Respiratory depression is a contraindication for dental treatment under general anaesthesia.

Table 13.5 Potential consequences of spinal cord injury

Level of injury	Motor loss	Sensory loss
C1 to C4 Quadriplegia	Paralysis of diaphragm, intercostal muscles with flaccid total paralysis below the neck	From the neck downwards
C5 to C8 Paraplegia	Paralysis of intercostals muscles below shoulders and upper arms	Arms, hands, chest, abdomen and lower limbs
T1 to T6	Paralysis below the mid chest	Below the mid chest
T7 to T12	Paralysis below waist	Below waist
T12 to L1	Paralysis in most leg muscles and pelvis	Lower abdomen and legs

13.13 Brain injury

It is estimated that a million people in the UK attend hospital each year as a result of a head injury[26]. The annual incidence is approximately 3 per 1,000 of the population. Of these, between 10 and 15 suffer a severe head injury. As with spinal injuries, common causes are RTAs (40% – 50%), domestic and industrial accidents (20% – 30%), sport and recreation (10% – 15%) and assaults (10%). Males are two to five times more likely to have a head injury than females. Cycling injuries account for approximately 20% of all head injuries to children.

The most visible signs of brain injury include coma, loss of power in limbs and speech impairment. However traumatic brain injury (TBI) causes numerous 'hidden disabilities' that result in changes in personality, thought and memory, and behaviour. Residual impairment depends upon the nature and severity of injury, speed and expertise in management and the individual's previous personality, ability and skills. Severe head injury can result in coma, a profound or deep state of unconsciousness. Up to 60% of all patients admitted to hospital in coma are alcoholics who have often had a head injury[27]. Persistent vegetative state (PVS), which sometimes follows coma, refers to a condition in which the individual has lost cognitive neurological function and awareness of the environment but retains non-cognitive function and a preserved sleep-wake cycle. There are normally less than 100 people in the UK with PVS at any one time.

Various problems may be encountered in people with brain injury (*Table 13.6*)

Table 13.6

Possible problems	Possible symptoms
Personality changes	Epilepsy
Depression	Changes in sexual drive
Memory loss and poor recall	Difficulty using hands and limbs
Frustration	Dizziness
Poor concentration and motivation	Dyspraxia
Mood changes	Sensory deprivation
Comprehension	Headaches
Inhibition	Weakness and paralysis
Tiredness and lethargy	

Traumatic brain injury (TBI) may be associated with other physical disabilities due to trauma. Diabetes may occur as a result of basal skull fractures or damage to the pituitary stalk. Brain injury can also result in a range of other medical complications. Many of the symptoms associated with TBI will also be found in other causes of acquired brain injuries.

During early management, the effects of nasal oxygen, mouth-breathing, intermittent suction of the airway, constant open mouth posture during intubation and restriction of oral nutrition will contribute to xerostomia. Oral health may be further complicated by therapeutic dehydration. In functional terms, skills that enable the individual to perform the activities of daily living may be lost. Self-care may be replaced by dependence even though there is no visible reason for this, and the image created in the lay-person's mind is of a learning disability. Coping with personality and behaviour changes creates stressful pressures on the head-injured person, their family and friends.

Severe physical or cognitive impairment will necessitate support for oral hygiene (Chapter 18). Visual neglect, when the individual is cognitively unaware of half the visual field or body, will affect oral hygiene. Transference of skills from the dominant hand will affect manual skills. Visual agnosia, defined as impaired object recognition, may be demonstrated by inability to recognise common objects such as a toothbrush and toothpaste. Memory loss may interfere with previously acquired skills, while cognitive impairment may lead to difficulty with the sequence of activities in simple tasks such as toothbrushing. These features may affect any person suffering from acquired brain injury.

Abnormal oral reflexes, lip biting, bruxism and rumination may result in severe dental or soft tissue trauma, and severe lip or tongue laceration[28]. Management options include monitoring lesions, smoothing sharp teeth, providing bite raising appliances or even extracting teeth. Various forms of appliance are described to help manage this difficult symptom[28,29].

Rehabilitation involves inter-disciplinary assessment, including rehabilitation medicine, neuropsychology, speech and language therapy, physiotherapy, occupational therapy, dietetics and of course family and carers, in order to develop individual goals for independence. The dental team needs to be involved in programmes that involve oral care skills. Regular domiciliary visits from a dental hygienist may be necessary to support family and carers in maintaining oral health. The primary care team should ensure that regular dental care can be accessed.

13.14 Epilepsy

Epilepsy is the term for a group of disorders characterised by repeated seizures that originate in the brain. A sudden, temporary interruption in some or all of the functions of nerve cells is the cause of a 'seizure' or 'fit'. Epilepsy is the second commonest neurological disorder, affecting around 1 in 200 adults and 1 in 100 children[30]. It is commoner in children and people with learning difficulties, and may present as a symptom of organic brain disease, as a consequence of brain injury, substance abuse or metabolic disorders. Epilepsy may take many forms and can be subdivided into different categories by cause and type of seizure. In idiopathic epilepsy, there is no clear cause and genetic factors may be responsible. Symptomatic epilepsy develops as a result of structural abnormality in the brain and is usually secondary to local or generalised brain disease. In cryptogenic epilepsy, no cause can be found but one is suspected. Seizures may be focal or generalised, and further subdivided into partial or complete, tonic-clonic, atonic, myoclonic, absence and nocturnal. The most recognised type of seizure is tonic-clonic or 'grand mal'. If a seizure is not self-limiting, lasts for more than five minutes or restarts, this is status epilepticus and requires urgent medical intervention.

Seizure control is achieved with anti-convulsant medication, with up to 70% becoming seizure free. Oral side-effects are listed in *Table 13.7*. Blood dyscrasias are reported side-effects; these may be reflected in the mouth. Oral side-effects of concurrent antipsychotic medication should also be considered. Phenytoin used to be one of the most effective drugs for seizure control; gross gingival hyperplasia was a frequent occurrence in people with a learning difficulty who were institutionalised (*Figure 11.2*). Gingival hyperplasia is sometimes associated with gingival tenderness. In the most severe cases, teeth may become submerged beneath the gingival overgrowth. There is now a much wider choice of anti-epileptic drugs that do not have this disfiguring side-effect; oral side-effects are always secondary to the importance of controlling seizures. However, gingival hyperplasia can largely be prevented by good plaque control.

Table 13.7 Side-effects of anti-convulsant medication

Drug	Side effect
Acetazolamide	Taste disturbance Stevens-Johnson syndrome
Carbamazepine	Stevens-Johnson syndrome Involuntary facial movements
Clobazam	Salivation changes
Clonazepam	Hypersalivation in infants
Ethosuximide	Gingival hyperplasia Stevens-Johnson syndrome Tongue swelling
Gabapentin	Pharyngitis Stevens-Johnson syndrome
Lamotrigine	Stevens-Johnson syndrome
Oxcarbazepine	Stevens-Johnson syndrome
Phenobarbitone	Bullous erythema multiforme (extremely rare)
Phenytoin	Gingival hyperlasia Stevens-Johnson syndrome
Sodium Valproate	Stevens-Johnson syndrome
Topiramate	Taste disorders

Accidental injury to teeth and soft tissues may occur during seizures, and there is a greater incidence of fractured or damaged teeth (*Figure 11.2*). Fragments of retained teeth and roots in bone or soft tissues may remain dormant and symptomless, but can cause acute pain and infection. They can be identified by x-ray. Bleeding tendencies are associated with sodium valproate, which may complicate extractions.

Dentures are not advised in people with severe epilepsy because of the risk of inhaling part of a fractured denture. Therefore it is particularly important to prevent tooth loss and the need for dentures. If dentures are required, it is advisable to consult the patient's neurologist about the risk of inhalation. Dentures constructed from radio-opaque acrylic permit identification on radiographs. Metal dentures are an alternative but each patient should be individually assessed. Treatment should ideally be provided during phases when seizures are infrequent. If treatment is required under general anaesthesia, it is essential that prescribed anti-epileptic medication is taken as normal.

13.15 Sensory impairment

There is very little published research on the oral health needs of people with sensory impairment. But it is possible to draw some conclusions from research into the social exclusion experienced by this very diverse population. The effects of sensory impairment are wide reaching. They include social, emotional, practical and information deficit.

13.16 Vision impairment

Vision impairment is generally equated with blindness but ranges from complete loss of vision to partial sightedness. 'Blind' means a high degree but not necessarily total loss, of vision. Profound blindness is the inability to distinguish fingers at a distance of three metres or less. Partial sight or 'severe low vision' is the inability to distinguish fingers at six metres or less. Few people classified as blind have no vision; a minority can distinguish light but nothing else. Some have no central vision; others have no lateral vision. For some people everything is a vague blur; others see a patchwork of blanks and defined areas. Visual impairment is largely an age-related problem; 90% of all people who are blind or partially sighted are over 60, a total of 2 million people whereas, only 8% of blind and partially sighted people are born with impaired vision[31], and 1 in 12 people over the age of 60 and 1 in 5 over 75 have a serious sight problem. Apart from congenital and age related causes, vision impairment can be caused by malnutrition, infection, medical conditions e.g. diabetes and trauma. Consequently, associated medical problems such as diabetes need consideration[32].

Apart from barriers to oral health associated with access and information deficit, oral hygiene may be inadequate in people with no visual feedback and oro-facial trauma may be more frequent due to falls. There is very little research on the oral health of people with vision impairment. Studies of younger people and adults report poorer levels of oral hygiene and more teeth extracted due to periodontal disease compared with sighted cohorts[33-35]. Teaching oral hygiene skills must take account of lack or restricted visual feedback and maximise the use of tactile skills[36]. The Touch Tooth Kit has been developed to teach oral hygiene skills to children with severe vision impairment[37]. Information should be available in a range of accessible formats to comply with the Disability Discrimination Act (1995)[38].

13.17 Hearing impairment

Many people experience hearing loss ranging from slight to profound deafness. About 8.7 million people in the UK, 1 in 7 of the total population and 1 in 5 adults – have hearing loss; the majority are over 50 years of age and 5.9 million people are thought to be sufficiently deaf or hard of hearing to be considered disabled under the 1995 Disability Discrimination Act[39]. Hearing loss is acquired or congenital. The commonest cause of acquired hearing loss is ageing. Rubella, mumps, meningitis and severe head injuries may also cause deafness. One to two children per thousand are born with significant, permanent deafness; of these, an estimated 50% are severely or profoundly deaf. Over 90% of deaf children are born to hearing parents.

Hearing impairment is classified as:

Mild hearing loss:	Difficulty following what is being said in groups or noisy situations.
Moderate hearing loss:	Difficulty following what is being said without a hearing aid, and particularly in a noisy situation.
Severe hearing loss:	Difficulty following what is being said even with a hearing aid.

People in all three categories come from very different cultures, and have a varied range of experiences and need for services[39]. The traditional definition of deafness as a medical condition consisting of an impaired sense of hearing has been countered by those who are born deaf or are prelingually deaf and use sign language. They have a different linguistic and cultural perspective which defines deafness as a way of life, with its own cultural identity and language. Disability resulting from hearing impairment is therefore seen in terms of social discrimination rather than an individual 'handicap'[40].

There are no specific oral and dental problems associated with hearing impairment, except in rare cases, when it is associated with congenital conditions such as Treacher Collins or rubella syndrome, learning disabilities or cardiac disease. In rubella syndrome, enamel defects may occur and bruxism (persistent tooth grinding) may be a feature. Sensitive and skilled communication may be necessary to teach oral hygiene skills and an understanding of the different communication modes, e.g. BSL interpreters, lip speaking, note taking and the use of deaf technology are essential in providing oral health care and complying with the DDA[38].

13.18 Dual sensory impairment

Dual sensory impairment does not necessarily mean total loss of vision and hearing but the combination of these impairments require special consideration. 'Deafblind' refers to a person when neither their sight nor their hearing can compensate for the impairment of the other sense, so that they cannot function either as a deaf person or as a blind person. The number of UK deafblind people has been estimated at 23,000 of which 15,000 are aged over 70 years of age[41]; their dental care requires an understanding of the various communication methods used.

13.19 Summary

This chapter summarises the most common causes of neurological and sensory impairment in adults, and their possible impact on oral health due to impairment or treatment. Many of the conditions described lead to an increased dependence for the activities of daily living, including oral hygiene. Oral health may deteriorate, reducing the potential for quality of life and increasing the possibility of crisis management for pain relief. To avoid this and reduce the burden on carers, referral for advice and treatment should be made as soon as possible after diagnosis. Guidance is available for health professionals who are in a prime position to initiate this process and provide informed advice and support[42].

References

1. Ford HL, Gerry L, Johnson M *et al.* A prospective study of the incidence, prevalence and mortality of multiple sclerosis in Leeds. *J Neurology* 2002 **249:** 260-265.

2. Multiple Sclerosis Society. What is MS? 2002. www.mssociety.org.uk

3. Bech E, Lycke J, Gadeberg P *et al.* A randomised, double-blind, placebo-controlled MRI study of anti-herpes virus therapy in MS. *Neurology* 2002 **58:** 31-36.

4. Symons AL, Bortolanza M, Godden S *et al.* A preliminary study into the dental health status of multiple sclerosis. *J Oral Med* 1993 **13:** 96-101.

5. Fiske J, Griffiths J, Thompson S. Multiple sclerosis and oral care. *Dent Update* 2002 **29:** 271-283.

6. Olaffson E, Benedikz J, Hauser WA. Risk of epilepsy in patients with multiple sclerosis: a population based study. *Epilepsia* 1999 **40:** 745-747.

7. McGrother CW, Dugmore CW, Phillips MJ *et al.* Multiple sclerosis, dental caries and fillings: a case-control study. *Br Dent J* 1999 **187:** 261-264.

8. Griffiths JE, Trimlett HJ. Dental status and barriers to care for adults with multiple sclerosis. *Int Dent J* 1996 **46:** 445.

9. American Dental Association. Don't remove amalgam fillings. *Lancet* 2002 **360:** 393.

10. Scully C, Cawson RA. Neurological disorders. In: *Medical Problems in Dentistry.* P336-373. Oxford: Butterworth-Heineman, 1998.

11. The Stroke Association. Stroke – questions and answers. Stroke Association. 2000. www.stroke.org.uk

12. Wright SM. Denture treatment for the stroke patient. *Br Dent J* 1997 **183:** 179-184.

13. Dicks JL, Banning J. Evaluation of calculus accumulation in tube-fed mentally handicapped patients: the effects of oral hygiene status. *Spec Care Dent* 1991 **11:** 104-106.

14. Jowett NI, Cabot LB. Patients with cardiac disease: considerations for the dental practitioner. *Br Dent J* 2000 **189:** 297-302.

15. Lockhart PB, Gibson J, Pond SH *et al.* Dental management considerations for the patient with an acquired coagulopathy. Part 2: Coagulopathies from drugs. *Br Dent J* 2003 **195:** 495-501.

16. Trigeminal Neuralgia Association. What is trigeminal neuralgia? www.tna-support.org accessed 2003

17. Huntington's Disease Association. Factsheets. http://www.had.org.uk accessed 2003.

18. Parkinson's Disease Association. www.parkinsons.org.uk accessed 2003.

19. Fiske J, Hyland K. Parkinson's diease and oral care. *Dent Update* 2002 **27:** 58-65.

20. Hyland K, Fiske J, Matthews N. Nutritional and dental health management in Parkinson's disease. *J Commun Nurs* 2000 **14:** 28-32.

21. Clifford TJ, Warsi MJ, Burnett CA *et al.* Burning mouth in Parkinson's disease sufferers. *Gerodontology* 1998 **15:** 73-78.

22. Spinal Injuries Association. Factsheets. 2001. www.sia.co.uk

23. Lancashire P, Jantzen J, Zach GA *et al*. The oral hygiene and gingival health of paraplegic inpatients – a cross-sectional survey. *J Clin Periodontol* 1997 **24**: 198-200.

24. Stiefel DJ, Truelove EL, Persson RS *et al*. A comparison of oral health in spinal cord injury and other disability groups. *Spec Care Dent* 1993 **13**: 229-235.

25. Bronte S. Oral health care for individuals with tetraplegia due to spinal cord injury – a pilot study. *J Disabil Oral Health* 2001 **2**: 30-36.

26. Headway. Head Injury - A Silent Epidemic. www.headway.org.uk accessed 2004

27. Scully C, Cawson RA. Maxillofacial trauma and head injury. In: *Medical Problems in Dentistry*. P454-469. Oxford: Butterworth-Heineman, 1998.

28. Millwood J, Fiske J. Lip-biting in patients with profound neuro-disability. *Dent Update* 2001 **28**: 105-108.

29. Griffiths JE. Preventing self-inflicted soft tissue trauma: a case report in an adult with severe neurological impairment. *J Disabil Oral Health* 2001 **2**: 27-29.

30. National Society for Epilepsy. Epilepsy: Information on seizures. 2002. www.epilepsynse.org.uk

31. Royal National Institute for the Blind. Factsheet. www.rnib.org.uk accessed 2002

32. Bell GW, Large DM, Barclay SC. Oral health care in diabetes mellitus. *Dent Update* 1999 **26**: 322-330.

33. Anaise JZ. Periodontal disease and oral hygiene in a group of blind and sighted teenagers in Israel. *J Dent Child* 1976 **7**: 353-356.

34. Greeley CB, Goldstein PA, Forrester DJ. Oral manifestations in a group of blind students. *J Dent Child* 1976 **43**: 39-42.

35. Campisi G, Cumbo V. A survey of dental-periodontal pathology in a sample of blind adult subjects. *Minerva Stomatol* 1994 **43**: 29-32.

36. O'Donnell D. Crosswaite MA. Dental health education for the visually impaired child. *Dent Health* 1991 **30**: 8-9.

37. Cleary JL, Valentine AD. The 'Touch Tooth' Kit. *Dent Practice* 1988 **26**: 1-3.

38. Disability Discrimination Act, 1995.

39. Robinson CA *et al*. Assessment and care management: the needs of older people with a sensory impairment. Final report to the Wales Office of Research and Development on behalf of the Welsh Assembly. Centre for Social Policy Research and Development., Bangor, 2001.

40. Young A, Ackerman J, Kyle J. *Looking on: Deaf people and the organisation of services*. Policy Press, University of Bristol, Joseph Rowntree Foundation, 1998.

41. Social Services Inspectorate. A sharper focus: Inspection of services for adults who are visually impaired or blind. 1998. Social Care Group, Department of Health.

42. Griffiths J. Guidelines for oral health care for people with a physical disability. *J Disabil Oral Health* 2002 **3**: 51-58.

Chapter 14

Impairment in adults - systemic disease

14.1 Introduction

Oral disease and discomfort may be the direct result of illness or secondary to its treatment. Conditions where general health is compromised by oral health are included in this chapter. There will inevitably be difficulties in classifying specific conditions into groups of impairments. This chapter will attempt to include some of the major conditions not yet covered in Section 3. Dental management may be complicated and pose a potential risk to health. Dental treatment may pose a serious health risk, particularly if a general anaesthetic is needed. To avoid crisis management, good preventive oral care including diet, good oral hygiene and regular dental attendance are therefore a priority.

14.2 Coronary heart disease

Coronary heart disease (CHD) is a largely preventable condition that is common in the UK and is frequently fatal. The death rate is higher than in many European countries and has fallen more slowly. In England it kills more than 110,000 people a year and about 300,000 people have a heart attack each year. It affects the unskilled male at more than three times the rate of those in managerial and professional occupations in terms of dying prematurely. Similarly, the wives of manual workers have more than twice the risk of being affected than the wives of managerial and professional workers of. Angina, heart attack and stroke are also more common in those with manual occupations. The death rate is higher for people born in the Indian sub-continent by 38% for males and 43% for women[1].

The major approach to reducing the impact of CHD is via a National Service Framework[1]. This brings together all members of the health care teams and social care with a clear plan to:

- Set national standards for prevention and treatment
- Recommend service models
- Suggest clinical audit and indicators to assess quality of prevention and treatment
- Set goals
- Provide examples of practical tools.

Risk factors for CHD

The major risk factors for CHD are:

- Smoking
- Excess alcohol
- Diabetes mellitus
- High cholesterol
- Family history of CHD
- Sedentary lifestyle
- Obesity.

In addition, there has been considerable research over the last ten years into the links between oral disease and CHD. Periodontal disease is a chronic infection and a possible source of infection, which can enter the circulation (bacteraemia). A recent review concluded that periodontal disease appears to be associated with a 19% increase in risk of future cardiovascular disease[2]. It is also clear that smoking is a cofactor in both periodontal disease and CHD[3].

A 'common risk factor' approach (See Chapter 19) to both CHD and oral health is a logical approach to prevention for both these common diseases. Promotion of a healthy diet, healthy lifestyle, good oral hygiene and smoking cessation are the principal components.

Cardiovascular diseases

There is a range of cardiovascular diseases that pose a risk for oral health, often as a result of the medications used. The following aspects of cardiovascular disease will affect dental treatment and careful medical history taking and treatment planning is needed:

- Chest pain
- Angina
- Myocardial infarction
- Hypertension
- Syncope
- Shortage of breath
- Rheumatic fever
- Infective endocarditis
- Cardiac arhythmia
- Cardiomyopathy
- Coronary artery bypass graft

- Valve replacements
- Congenital disorders
- Cardiac transplants
- Venous/lymphatic disorders[4].

For these aspects of cardiovascular disease, effective dental treatment and prevention will often involve collaboration with the wider health care team. Dental treatment will usually avoid general anaesthetics and the use of adrenaline containing local anaesthetic. Timing for dental treatment may be affected by the phase of the disease, e.g. delaying treatment until three months post myocardial infarction. Antibiotic cover for some forms of dental treatment may be needed in many conditions, e.g. Rheumatic fever, to prevent infective endocarditis.

Oral side-effects of medications used in cardiovascular disease

Certain groups of medications used in the treatment of cardiovascular disease have a specific side effect on oral health. For further details see Chapter 8.

Beta blockers

These are used in the control of high blood pressure and cardiac failure. Side effects include xerostomia (dry mouth) and lichenoid reactions.

Vasodilators

This group of drugs is used to decrease the blood pressure by dilating veins. Calcium antagonists are used to control coronary and peripheral blood vessel dilation. Oral side effects include gingival hyperplasia.

Immunosuppressives

These drugs are used post-cardiac transplant to reduce rejection of the new organ. Oral side effects include infection by Candida (*Figure 2.5 - 2.6*) and gingival hyperplasia (*Figure 8.3*).

14.3 Blood disorders

Abnormalities in the blood can be classified into disorders of:

- Red blood cells
- White blood cells
- Platelets
- Clotting and bleeding disorders.

It is important to detect blood disorders during the taking of a medical history prior to commencing dental treatment. Blood disorders can cause excessive bleeding following surgical procedures and healing may be affected. The choice of local anaesthetic and technique may also be affected. There is a need for effective prevention to minimise dental interventions that often pose a risk for people with blood disorders.

Red blood cells- anaemia

Anaemia may be caused by one of a number of factors:

- Excessive haemorrhage
- Abnormalities in red cell formation- aplastic anaemia
- Increased red cell destruction- haemolytic anaemia.

The causes of anaemia include:

- Excessive haemorrhage: menorrhagia, gastro-intestinal ulcer/carcinoma, trauma
- Malabsorbtion syndromes
- Pregnancy
- Nutritional deficiencies- iron, vitamin B12, folate
- Drug induced anaemia
- Malignancies
- Secondary to chronic disease
- Infection: malaria
- Inherited conditions- sickle cell disease, thalassaemias.

The oral signs and symptoms of anaemia include:

- Generalised soreness of the soft tissues
- Persistent ulceration
- Red, smooth tongue
- Candidal infection and angular cheilitis
- Abnormalities in taste sensation.

White blood cells

White blood cell disorders can include:

- Reduced numbers (leucopaenia)
- Increased numbers (leucocytosis) - a feature of leukaemia
- Malignancy (see Chapter 16).

Leucopaenia

This may be the result of HIV infection or early stages of leukaemia, or may be due to drug therapy. The clinical condition is known as aganulocytosis and causes an increased susceptibility to infection and oral ulceration.

Platelets

There may be decreased numbers of platelets or failure in function. This can produce bleeding following dental surgery. Platelet function can be affected by drugs e.g. aspirin.

Clotting and bleeding disorders

These disorders may be related to:

- Inherited-Haemophilia- Von Willebrands disease, Christmas disease
- Anti-coagulant drugs-Warfarin, Aspirin, Heparin.

Dental treatment will need to be planned in conjunction with the haematology team to replace missing clotting factors in inherited disease. There are increased numbers of people taking anti-coagulants to reduce the risk of stroke. Dental surgery needs careful planning after assessing their bleeding time and careful control of post-operative bleeding[5].

14.4 Respiratory disorders

Respiratory disorders are common, and in common with other systemic conditions, they can affect the way that dental treatment is carried out. There is an increased risk with general anaesthesia, sedation and side effects with some of the medications. The increased risk associated with dental care raises the importance of effective prevention. Respiratory diseases will always be affected by smoking, therefore this common risk factor for oral disease should also be addressed by the dental team.

Asthma

Asthma is a generalised airway obstruction which leads to the characteristic wheeze following muscle contractions in the bronchus. The condition is provoked by contact with allergens, stress and effort. Infrequent attacks are controlled by ventolin inhalers, which act as a bronchodilator. More frequent attacks are controlled by regular use of salbutamol or inhaled steriods.

The oral side effects of long-term treatment are a dry mouth and increased risk of candidal infection.

Chronic obstructive airways disease

This condition combines chronic bronchitis and emphysema and is a common smoking related disease. There is a combination of chronic sputum production and dilation and destruction of the bronchioles. Treatment involves bronchodilators and antibiotics. Steriods are also used which can affect the timing of dental treatment[6].

Tuberculosis

Tuberculosis is an infection from *Mycobacterium tuberculosis* which has increased in prevalence in recent years. It is seen in immunocompromised people with HIV and in immigrants from non-industrialised countries who are malnourished. Lesions can occasionally be seen on the tongue. The condition is infectious when active which can affect the timing of dental treatment. It is treated by a combination of specific antibiotics (See also, Chapter 15).

Cystic fibrosis

Cystic fibrosis is a common, inherited disease seen in 1:2,000 live births. The condition affects the lungs and digestive system. Respiratory infections are common and require prolonged antibiotic therapy. Malnutrition is a problem of impaired digestion and there is a risk of diabetes mellitus and liver disease. The oral features include enlargement of the salivary glands, enamel hypoplasia and delayed eruption. Dietary supplements high in sugar are often used but a high caries rate is not seen, thought to be due to the long-term antibiotic usage. Higher levels of calculus are seen which is thought to be due to a high calcium content of saliva in this condition[7].

14.5 Gastrointestinal disease

Gastrointestinal diseases can have oral signs and the sequelae can have an effect on oral health. The dental management of people with gastrointestinal disease can be affected in the timing and choice of anaesthesia.

Some of the aspects of GI disease include:

- Anaemia
- Gastric reflux
- Vomiting
- Dysphagia (difficulty swallowing)
- Cervical node enlargement
- Facial and labial swelling in Crohn's disease.

Oral aspects of GI disease include:

- Oral ulceration
- Glossitis
- Burning mouth
- Angular cheilitis.

Side effects of some of drugs used in GI disease include:

- Candidal infections following extensive broad spectrum antibiotics for gastric ulcer treatment
- Oral irritation from pancreatic supplements
- Xerostomia from proton pump inhibitors.

14.6 Liver disease

There are few oral features in relation to liver disease. The common signs include jaundice, Dupuytren's contracture and finger clubbing. There may be a bleeding tendency, and intolerance to drugs used in dental care can affect dental management. Hepatitis requires extra care in cross-infection control (See Chapter 15).

14.7 Renal disease

Oral features occur only in the less common renal disorders. Children with chronic renal failure may have delayed eruption, malocclusions and enamel defects. Aspects of renal disease include:

- Anaemia
- Reduced salivary flow
- Keratin deposits (white patches)
- Oral infections in immunosupressed people after transplants
- Gingival hyperlasia following cyclosporin therapy.

Long term steriod therapy will also affect dental management[9].

14.8 Endocrine system disorders

The endocrine system consists of the group of glands that produce hormones. The commonest disorder is diabetes. Other disorders include:

- Thyroid gland disorders. Hypothyroidism can reduce the immune response and oral candidal infections may be seen.
- Oral contraceptives - may have reduced effect with antibiotics and increase gingivitis.
- Adrenal gland disorders. Excess production in Cushing's disease and Cushing's syndrome. Decreased production in Addison's disease, which requires replacement sterioids for surgical dental treatment.
- Parathyroid gland disorders. Hyperparathyroidism (excess production) may present with oral granulomas. Hypothryroidsism following surgery to the glands leads to bone resorption.
- Pituitary gland disorders. Increased growth hormone production causes acromegaly with increased growth of mandible, facial bones and hands.
- Diabetes insipidus - reduced anti-diuretic hormone can follow pituitary gland tumour or injury. Features include high fluid intake and urine production and xerostomia[10].

Diabetes mellitus

Diabetes mellitus is commonly referred to as 'diabetes' and is a chronic and progressive disease that affects children, young people and adults of all ages. Diabetes comprises a group of disorders with many different causes, all of which are characterised by a raised blood glucose level. The condition is increasing and around 1.3 million people in England are currently diagnosed with diabetes, in addition to many hundreds of thousands who may have Type 2 diabetes without yet knowing it.

- In Type 1 diabetes, (15% of cases) the pancreas is no longer able to produce insulin. Daily injections of insulin are required in order to maintain blood glucose within certain limits, which will require adjustments in diet and lifestyle.

- Type 2 diabetes, (85% of cases) the insulin producing cells are not able to produce enough for the body's needs. The majority of people with Type 2 diabetes also have some degree of insulin resistance. People with Type 2 diabetes need to adjust their diet and their lifestyle. Many are overweight or obese and will be advised to lose weight.

The incidence of diabetes is increasing in all age groups:

- Type 1 diabetes is increasing in children, particularly in under fives
- Type 2 diabetes is increasing across all groups, including children and young people, and particularly among black and minority ethnic groups.

Diabetes can result in premature death, ill health and disability via:

- Renal failure
- Neuropathy
- Vascular disease
- Ocular disease
- Cardiovascular disease[11].

People with well-controlled diabetes have no specific oral features. If poorly controlled, oral health may be affected by xerostomia, delayed healing, susceptibility to oral infections and periodontal disease. There is emerging research that links obesity to an increased prevalence of periodontal disease[12].

14.9 Summary

There are numerous rare conditions that may compromise oral health. This chapter has summarised the most significant non-malignant medical conditions. For most of the conditions, an avoidance of dental treatment under general anaesthesia is a priority. Basic oral prevention to reduce plaque levels, access to fluoride and a diet low in extrinsic sugars is important. Regular dental attendance for preventive advice and treatment to avoid crisis management will make an important contribution to the maintenance of health.

References

1. National Service Framework for Coronary Heart Disease. Executive Summary. 2000. http://www.doh.gov.uk
2. Janket SJ, Baird AE, Chuang SK *et al.* Meta-analysis of periodontal disease and risk of coronary heart disease and stroke. *Oral Surg Oral Med Oral Path* 2003 **95**: 559-569.
3. Hyman JJ, Winn DM, Reid BC. The role of cigarette smoking in the association between periodontal disease and coronary heart disease. *J Periodontol* 2002 **73**: 998-994.
4. Greenwood M, Meechan JG. General medicine and surgery for dental practitioners. Part 1: Cardiovascular system. *Br Dent J* 2003 **194**: 538.
5. Greenwood M, Meechan JG. General medicine and surgery for dental practitioners. Part 9: Haematology and patients with bleeding disorders. *Br Dent J* 2003 **195**: 306-310.
6. Greenwood M, Meechan JG. General medicine and surgery for dental practitioners. Part 2: Respiratory system. *Br Dent J* 2003 **194**: 593-598.

7. Narang A, Maguire A, Nunn JH *et al.* Oral health and related factors in cystic fibrosis and other chronic respiratory disorders. *Arch Disease Child* 2003 **88:** 702-707.

8. Greenwood M, Meechan JG. General medicine and surgery for dental practitioners. Part 3: Gastrointestinal system. *Br Dent J.* 2003 **194:** 659-663.

9. Greenwood M, Meechan JG. General medicine and surgery for dental practitioners. Part 7: Renal disorders. *Br Dent J.* 2003 **195:** 181-184.

10. Greenwood M, Meechan JG. General medicine and surgery for dental practitioners. Part 6: The endocrine system. *Br Dent J.* 2003 **195:** 129-133.

11. National Service Framework for Diabetes. Executive Summary. 2002. http://www.doh.gov.uk

12. Al-Zahrani MS, Bissada NF, Borawskit EA. Obesity and periodontal disease in young, middle-aged and older adults. *J Periodontol* 2003 **74:** 610-615.

Chapter 15

Impairment - oral infections and related conditions

15.1 Introduction

The mouth contains a vast number of organisms, many of which are normally non-pathogenic but can become pathogenic when the immune defences are weakened. An example is *Candida Albicans*, which produces candidiasis, or thrush, often an indicator of underlying systemic disease.

Other oral infections may include:

- HIV/AIDS
- Herpes viruses
- Hepatitis viruses
- Syphilis and other sexually transmitted diseases
- Tuberculosis
- Prions.

Transmission between individual patients, with the health care professional acting as a passive vector, is of particular importance for older or other compromised groups. An example is the *methicillin resistant Staphylococcus Aureus* (MRSA). This bacterium is readily transmitted via hand, nasal or oral contact and can produce a life-threatening systemic infection[1].

15.2 Candidiasis

Oral candidiasis (*Figures 2.5-2.6, 15.1-15.2*) is a common fungal infection, which is usually considered opportunistic with the presence of other factors including:

- Age: very young or very old
- Pregnancy
- Local trauma due to ill-fitting dentures
- Antibiotic therapy, particularly broad spectrum
- Corticosteriods, both systemic and via inhalers
- Malnutrition
- Endocrine disorders
- Malignancies including blood disorders
- Immune defects including HIV/AIDS
- Xerostomia.

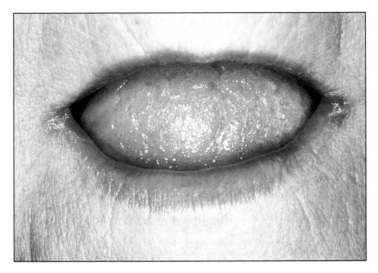

Figures 15.1 Candida associated angular cheilitis

It is the commonest infection in the mouth of individuals aged 70 and over, and wearing dentures strongly increases the candida oral population[2]. Oral candidiasis is the most common opportunistic infection among people with HIV[3], although the prevalence is reducing following the introduction of antiviral therapies[4].

Types of oral candidiasis

There are four distinct presentations of the condition. To obtain a definitive diagnosis a biopsy or smear test is required. Drug-resistant strains can also be identified.

Pseudomembranous candidiasis (thrush)

In this variant there are white meshes and patches on the mucous membranes of the cheek, tongue, or floor of the mouth. The pseudomembrane (false membrane) can be wiped off to leave a bleeding surface.

Atrophic candidiasis

Atrophic candidiasis is a more chronic form commonly seen in denture wearers. The reddened painless area is usually limited to the oral mucosa covered by the denture. Red patches can also be observed on the tongue and buccal mucosa.

Chronic hyperplastic candidiasis

This presents as white patches, nodules or patches with red flecks in various sites in the mouth. The lesions should be excised and biopsied as there may be early signs of malignancy.

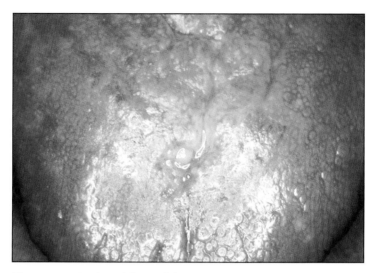

Figures 15.2 Oral candidiasis of the tongue

Candida associated angular cheilitis

This variant presents as chronic ulcers and cracking in the corners of the mouth (*Figure 15.1*). In the denture wearer it may be caused by worn dentures leading to overclosure of oral musculature. Ulcers may be secondarily infected from bacteria on the skin or nostrils. Angular cheilitis in younger groups is also commonly seen in people living with HIV.

Treatment of oral candidiasis

There are several anti-fungal drugs available which can be applied topically or systemically. The most effective topical treatment uses Fluconazole, which is rinsed and then swallowed. In the case of denture wearers it is important to effectively clean the dentures to remove a pool of infection which can re-infect. Anti-fungal drug resistance is common among people with advanced AIDS[5].

15.3   Human immunodeficiency virus (HIV)

Infection with HIV causes a disease that suppresses the immune system and leaves the individual susceptible to a wide variety of infections. Infection with HIV is also linked to a group of otherwise rare tumours. The condition, acquired immune deficiency syndrome (AIDS), is unusual in that it is a form of immunodeficiency that is transmissible.

Since the 1980s the impact of AIDS as a global epidemic has become apparent. Some of the key figures, which demonstrate the impact of the disease, include:

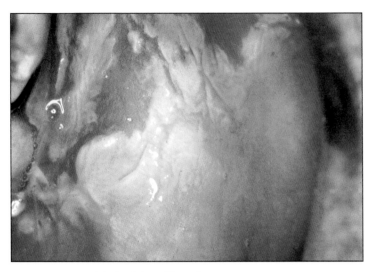

Figures 15.3 Oral leukoplakia of buccal mucosa

- Number of people living with HIV in 2003: 37 million adults and 2.5 million children
- Number of people infected with HIV in 2003: 4.2 million adults and 700,000 children
- AIDS deaths in 2003: 2.5 million adults and 500,000 children
- Total number of AIDS deaths until the end of 2001: 21.8 million including 4.3 million children6.

The number of people living with HIV in high-income countries is continuing to rise due to the introduction of highly active antiretroviral therapy (HAART). In Western Europe, North America, Australia and New Zealand, the impact of AIDS is estimated to be:

- 1.6 million people living with HIV
- 80,000 newly infected in 2003
- 18,000 deaths from AIDS.

There is evidence that changes in lifestyle and other preventive actions are not affecting the rising infection rate[6]. The impact of this global pandemic will mean that the primary health care team will have increasing contact with people living with HIV.

Transmission of HIV

HIV has been detected in blood, plasma, semen, saliva, tears and cerebrospinal fluid. The main route of transmission is via sexual intercourse. The are a number of risk groups in society whose lifestyles are more likely to lead to transmission but with the increase in infection it is not possible to identify all those individuals at risk.

Although HIV can be detected in the saliva of infected individuals it appears to be of low infectivity compared to other body fluids. However, all health care workers should still maintain consistent infection control measures with all body fluids.

Oral manifestations of HIV infection

Oral manifestations of HIV are seen in approximately 30-80% of the affected population[7]. Oral lesions are linked to the activity of the disease and the level of circulating virus. The types of manifestations fall into the four groups shown in *Table 15.1*[8].

Table 15.1

Type of lesion	Includes
Neoplastic	Kaposi's sarcoma Lymphoma
Bacterial	Linear gingival erythema Necrotising ulcerative periodontitis Tuberculosis Mycobacterium avium complex Bacillary angiomatosis
Viral	Herpes simplex Herpes zoster Cytomegalovirus ulcers Hairy leukoplakia Warts
Fungal	Candidiasis Angular chelitis Histoplasmosis Cryptococcosis

With many of the oral conditions acting as 'markers' for the conversion of HIV infection to AIDS, early recognition and treatment can reduce morbidity. The prevalence of oral related aspects of HIV has changed since the introduction of HAART. There is evidence that some of the lesions, e.g. hairy leukoplakia, have reduced but this reduction is not seen across all the manifestations[9].

Oral health care for people with HIV/AIDS

Control and prevention of oral disease is important for people with HIV/AIDS infection as their deficient immune system will raise the severity and duration of any oral conditions. Planning dental treatment for people in the more advanced stage of AIDS will need to be done in collaboration with their medical team. Complex dental treatment plans, particularly those involving extractions need to be considered in relation to the person's immunological status. There are few risks of complications of dental treatment with the exception of the effects of anaemia and bleeding times. People with HIV and AIDS may be receiving a complex range of drug therapies that will result in xerostomia.

15.4 Herpes virus infection

The commonest infections encountered in this group include:

- Herpes simplex type I virus
- Herpes simplex type II virus
- Varicella zoster virus
- Epstein barr virus
- Cytomegalovirus
- Human herpes virus 6
- Human herpes virus 7
- Human herpes virus 8.

These viruses produce a variety of infectious conditions and may also be associated with HIV/AIDS and other underlying systemic conditions.

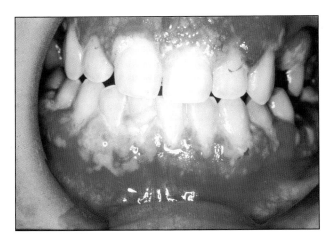

Figure 15.4
The oral effects
of Herpes
Stomatitis

Herpes simplex type I virus (HSV-1)

The initial infection with HSV-1 occurs in early childhood and the commonest site of infection is via small abrasions in the oral mucosa. The oral condition, gingivostomatitis, can vary in severity from mildly irritating vesicles to more severe oral ulceration, blood encrusted lips and a raised temperature. Vesicles can break down and ulcerate and there is a risk of secondary bacterial infection. Healing is more rapid if the condition is treated with systemic acyclovir, a specific anti-viral agent. Once ulcers are established, care of the mouth involves the use of antiseptic mouthwashes (chlorhexidine) and oral hygiene measures. Lesions tend to persist for 10-14 days and heal without scarring. They are very infectious and there is a risk of spreading the infection to fingers, nose, eyes or genitals.

After the primary infection, latent HSV-1 persists in the nerve ganglion and can reactivate causing a recurrent condition in 15-20% of cases known as Recurrent Herpes Labialis. These lesions, also known as 'cold sores' occur on the lips or peri-orbital tissues. They are triggered by a number of factors including:

- Trauma
- Sunlight
- Stress
- Systemic upset.

The lesion starts with a prickling sensation, followed by discrete vesicles that break down to form the distinctive crusted lesion that lasts 7-10 days. Treatment should be started early and consists of applications of topical acyclovir five times a day. The 'experienced' sufferer is usually aware of the early symptoms. Severe cases may require systemic acyclovir, particularly in the immuno-suppressed. HSV-1 is present in saliva and mucosal membranes throughout the infection; care should be taken by health workers to avoid infection. Direct infection of cutaneous sites such as fingers or toes can lead to a lesion known as an 'herpetic whitlow[10].

Herpes simplex type II virus (HSV-2)
This variety of herpes simplex virus can cause oral infection but is mostly associated with genital infections[11].

Varicella zoster virus
This member of the herpes group (VZV) is named after Varicella, the primary VZV infection, chickenpox and Zoster, another name for shingles, which is the reactivation of the latent virus. The primary infection, chicken pox, is a common feature of childhood. Up to 90% of young adults in temperate countries will contract the condition that is highly infectious.

The condition is composed of headaches, fever and the characteristic skin lesions, which can be seen intra-orally.

The reactivated condition, known as 'shingles', arises as the VZV is latent in the nerve ganglia of the sensory and spinal nerves. The initial symptoms are pain followed by patches of ulceration. Treatment consists of pain relief and systemic acyclovir therapy. Postherpetic neuralgia may develop in up to a third of patients due to direct nervous tissue damage.

Epstein barr virus (EBV)
Infection with EBV occurring in early childhood is via saliva and results in a primary infection that is asymptomatic. A degree of protection against re-infection follows. If infection is delayed until adolescence the EBV infection gives rise to infectious mononucleosis or 'glandular fever'. A long-standing fever, pharyngeal inflammation and oral ulcerations are often seen. In more severe cases the liver and spleen are affected. Oral care consists of limiting secondary infection with oral care and antiseptic mouthwash.

EBV is also associated with a range of other conditions including:

- Endemic Burkitt's lymphoma (equatorial Africa)
- Undifferentiated nasopharyngeal carcinoma (southern China)
- EBV associated oral hairy leukoplakia in people with HIV/AIDS.

Cytomegalovirus
Infection with this herpes virus can occur postnatal via saliva or be acquired congenitally. The congenital infection can result in foetal damage and subsequent deafness or learning disability. The acquired infection is usually asymptomatic but can present as a glandular fever like illness. Re-infection and recurrent infection can occur in immunosupressed people and produce an hepatitis like illness.

Human herpes virus 6 and 7
These two herpes viruses can be transmitted via saliva. Infection is often asymptomatic but can present as a fever with a rose pink rash.

Human herpes virus 8
This herpes virus is linked with Karposi's sarcoma, the most common neoplasm in people with AIDS[12].

15.5 Sexually transmitted diseases (STDs)

The most common STDs, syphilis and gonorrhoea, both have oral manifestations that pose an infection risk for the health worker. One study reported up to 50% of lesions in the oral and pharyngeal mucosa[13].

15.6 Tuberculosis (TB)

Tuberculosis is an infectious disease, which most commonly affects the lungs but can also present with oral lesions. It is not a highly infectious condition and usually requires prolonged close contact with an infectious person. It is a global problem; cases in England and Wales have increased 27% in the last decade. Apart from those living in poverty and recent immigrants, HIV infection is a well-recognised risk factor for TB. TB can normally be controlled but drug-resistant tuberculosis is an increasing problem[14].

Orally transmitted infections

There are a number of important infective conditions, which do not have any specific oral manifestations. They do, however, pose an infection risk for the health care worker both for themselves and for other people in their care. Some of the important conditions include:

- Hepatitis
- MRSA
- Pneumonia
- CJD

15.7 Hepatitis

This blood borne infection has no oral lesions but remains important for the health worker involved in oral care because of the risk of transmission due to the presence of the virus in saliva. There are three main variants, A, B & C. Hepatitis B (HBV) is the most infective and robust and poses a challenge for cross infection control. The majority of people infected with HBV are asymptomatic and may be unaware of their carrier status. There are certain groups whose occupation or lifestyles can render them a high risk for HBV including:

- Health care staff, particularly those involved with drug dependency, haemodialysis and multiply transfused patients
- Laboratory staff in blood banks and pathology laboratories
- Asylum seekers
- People living and working in institutions and prisons

- High risk lifestyles including intravenous drug use
- Immunocompromised patients
- Long term travellers from low to high prevalence areas
- Partners and close relatives of the above.

In practice it should be assumed that every patient is a potential carrier and universal standards of cross infection control should be followed with all patients[15].

15.8 Multi-resistant staphylococcus aureus (MRSA)

Susceptibility to MRSA is linked to age and a number of other risk factors such as surgery, invasive devices and procedures. It is mostly of concern in hospitals and Intensive Care Units, operating theatres and surgical wards. It is considered less of a risk in community clinical practice. There are many different strains of MRSA but there is no evidence that it poses a risk to healthy people including healthcare workers and their families. Oral care is possible in units in which it is endemic by following a high standard of infection control[16].

15.9 Pneumonia

There is evidence emerging of the link between aspiration pneumonia and oral risk factors. Anaerobic bacteria from periodontal pockets have been isolated from infected lungs. This further highlights the need for improving oral hygiene amongst at risk people including older people and those living in long term care facilities[17].

15.10 Creutzfeldt-Jakob Disease (CJD)

This fatal condition is caused by prions, which are mutated proteins. The condition, also known as Transmissible spongiform encephalitis, which describes the actual disease, does not have any specific oral manifestations. There is a potential risk of a health worker becoming infected via accidental abrasion of an infected person's lingual tonsils or via needlestick injury with infected instruments. There are particular procedures regarding handling and disposal of instruments according to the risk status of infected people and their families. Although at 2003, there have only been a total of 900 confirmed deaths from CJD it is anticipated that numbers will rise over the coming decades[18].

15.11 Good practice guidelines for oral care

There are good practice universal protection guidelines, which should be utilised by all health care staff providing oral care.

• Immunisation
All clinical staff should be vaccinated against the common illnesses. For staff directly involved in the clinical aspects of oral care this should include Hepatitis B. Regular monitoring to ensure ongoing protection should also be undertaken.

• Medical history
Regular updating of the medical history will alert to the possibility of being in a high-risk group and the changing health status.

• Hand protection
Effective hand protection is fundamental to infection control. This includes effective hand washing and the wearing of gloves as a single use item for each patient. To ensure the effectiveness of washing, all jewellery should be removed, and cuts and abrasions covered with adhesive dressings.

• Eye protection and face masks
The eyes should be protected against foreign bodies, splatter and aerosols produced during oral care. Masks do not confer complete microbiological protection and should be changed between patients.

• Disposal of waste
Disposable products should be used wherever possible. For providing routine oral care for patients, toothbrushes provided should be regarded as single use items. Adequate provision should be made for the disposal of clinical waste including sharps and needles in safe containers.

• Surfaces
Wherever possible, disposable trays and covers should be used. Surfaces should be cleaned between patients with a detergent and disinfectant.

• Decontamination of instruments
Contaminated instruments should be cleaned by hand, ultrasonic bath or washer/disinfector and, when clean, autoclaved.

• Infection control policy and procedures
All members of the health care team should be trained in infection control and be aware of the procedures in the policy including how to deal with spillage and inoculation injuries.

For more information see the British Dental Association Advice Sheet 'A12' Infection Control in Dentistry[19].

References

1. Staat, RH, Stewart AV, Stewart JF. MRSA: an important consideration for geriatric dentistry practitioners. *Spec Care Dent* 1991 **11**: 197-199.

2. Rothan-Tondeur ML, Pialleport T, Meaume S *et al.* Prevalence of oropharyngeal candidiasis in geriatric in-patients. *J Amer Geriatrics Soc* 2001 **49**: 1741-1742.

3. Dodd CI *et al.* Oral candidiasis in HIV infection: pseudomembraneous and erythemaous candidiasis show similar rates of progression to AIDS. *AIDS* 1991 **5**: 1339.

4. Candidiasis. P4 Aidsmap. www.aidsmap.com

5. Candidiasis. P3 Aidsmap. www.aidsmap.com

6. Global statistical information & tables. www.avert.org

7. Reznik DA, O'Daniels C. Oral Manifestations of HIV/AIDS in the HAART era. Oral Manifestations and Dental Care Issues for Health Professionals. www.hivdent.org

8. Greenspan D, Greenspan JS. Oral Manifestations of HIV Infection. Oral Manifestations and Dental Care Issues for Health Professionals. www.hivdent.org

9. Patton LL, McKaig R, Strauss *et al.* Changing prevalence of oral manifestations of HIV in the era of protease inhibitor therapy. *Oral Surg Oral Med Oral Radiol Endod* 2000 **90**: 299-304.

10. Raborn GW, Grace M. Herpes Simplex Type 1 Orofacial Infections. *J of IHMF* 1999 **6**: 8-12.

11. Stanberry LR, Rosenthal SL. The Epidemiology of Herpes Simplex Virus infections in adolescents. *J of IHMF* 1999 **6**: 12-16.

12. Stanberry LR. Herpes virus: agents of acute and chronic disease. *J of IHMF* 2001 **8**: 59.

13. Melnichenko EM, Gusakovskaia ZhS. The characteristics of the manifestation of syphilis on the mucosa of the mouth and orophayrnx. *Stomatologiia* 2000 **79**: 53-55.

14. The Prevention and Control of Tuberculosis in the UK. Dept of Health. 1998.

15. Guidance for Clinical Health Workers: Protection Against Infections with Blood-borne Infections. Dept of Health. www.open.gov.uk/doh/chcguid1.ht

16. MRSA Policy. Gwent Healthcare NHS Trust. 2003.

17. Mojon P. Oral health and respiratory infection. *J Canadian Dent Assoc* 2002 **68**: 340-345.

18. Risk Assessment for vCJD and Dentistry. Dept of Health. www.doh.gov.uk/cjd/dentistryrisk/index.htm

19. Infection Control in Dentistry. Advice Sheet A12. London: BDA, 2003.

Chapter 16

Impairment - malignant disease and its treatment

16

16.1 Introduction

In the United Kingdom there are almost 250,000 new cases of cancer in adults and approximately 1,200 new cases of childhood cancer each year[1]. Advances in medicine have led to the development of new treatments for malignant disease. Early diagnosis and treatment can improve life expectancy. Changes in lifestyle and a greater focus on positive health by many groups in society, particularly in diet, have led to declines in some cancers. However, treatment regimes can involve painful and distressing side effects in addition to the emotional aspects of coping with cancer. The immunosuppressive aspects of cancer treatments can lead to increased susceptibility to infection. The oral cavity provides a pool of opportunistic infection, which may lead to life-threatening systemic infection. Up to 90% of children with cancer will have oral problems which can have long term effects[2].

This chapter concentrates on aspects of:

- Leukaemia and its oro-dental manifestations
- Oral cancer
- Oral aspects of treatment:
    - chemotherapy
    - radiotherapy
    - bone marrow transplantation
    - immunosuppressive therapy
    - surgery

Oral care for people within these groups is described, based on a comprehensive clinical pathway for the Oral Management of Oncology Patients Requiring Radiotherapy, Chemotherapy and Bone Marrow Transplantation[3].

16.2 Leukaemia

Leukaemia is the collective term for a group of progressively malignant blood disorders characterised by large numbers of abnormal white blood cells. In a single year in England there were nearly 6,000 cases diagnosed, of which over 300 were children[4]. Leukaemias are classified as acute and chronic and by the type of white blood cell: myeloid or lymphoblast. The acute variants have more immature or primitive white cells. Acute leukaemias are the commonest childhood cancer.

Symptoms of leukaemia which affect oral health include:

- Increased susceptibility to infection
- Bruising
- Bleeding tendencies
- Anorexia leading to poor nutritional status.

The oral signs and symptoms of leukaemia include:

- Pale soft tissues
- Gingival bleeding
- Gingival swelling (red, soft or spongy)
- Bruising
- Ulceration
- Swollen tonsils
- Swollen parotid salivary glands
- Infections including:
  Candidiasis (*Figures 2.5, 2.6, 15.1, 15.2*)
  Fungal infections
  Herpes virus (*Figure 15.4*)

Acute lymphoblastic and myeloblastic leukaemia produce a similar clinical picture. Variations occur in the different types with gingival swelling commonest in myeloblastic leukaemia. Treatment with cytotoxics causes further complications

16.3 Oral malignancy and maxillofacial surgery

Oral cancer, which includes oral, lip, salivary gland and pharyngeal tissues is one of the group of cancers with approximately 4,000 new cases per year (see Section 1.6). In the UK there are about 2,000 new cases per year but they may be under-reported by up to 25%. Despite progress in cancer diagnosis and treatment during the last decades, the prognosis of oral malignancies remains poor with a five-year survival rate of less than 55%. This poor prognosis has not changed over the past few decades. Oral cancer kills at least 1,400 people each year in England and Wales; nearly two thirds of patients with this cancer will die of their disease[5]. Common sites for oral malignancies include the floor of the mouth, border of the tongue and the lips. The commonest type is squamous cell carcinoma. Secondaries from other sites may affect the jaws and rarer malignancies may occur. Although rare, lymphomas affect the salivary glands, in particular the minor salivary glands.

Diagnosis and treatment are usually carried out by a specialist team including, maxillofacial surgeons, head and neck surgeons, radiation and medical oncologists. Treatment may consist of radiotherapy, chemotherapy and surgery. Surgery usually involves radical excision into healthy tissue beyond the margins of the lesion. Complex maxillofacial reconstruction and prostheses may be necessary to restore facial tissues and reduce disfigurement. Bone grafts may be required to restore the mandible. Support and counselling may be needed to help the person cope with psychological aspects of disfigurement. Some of the other complications include:

- Acute oral mucositis
- Xerostomia
- Speech and swallowing difficulties
- Nutritional problems.

16.4 Other malignancies

It is beyond the scope of this book to discuss this vast and complex area. Secondary lesions from breast, lung, thyroid, kidney, stomach and prostate may occur in the mouth, the jaws being the most frequent site. Systemic effects of malignancy may also present in the mouth. Treatments for malignancy have the potential to seriously affect oral health. These treatments include chemotherapy, radiotherapy and immunosuppressants.

16.5 Chemotherapy

Oral side effects of cytotoxics may exacerbate oral symptoms including:

- Ulceration
- Lip cracking
- Gingival swelling
- Bleeding
- Salivary gland pain
- Infections- particularly candidosis
- Xerostomia
- Pigmentation.

16.6 Radiotherapy

Radiation affecting the head and neck contributes to a number of oral complications. The degree of oral involvement depends on the type, dose and duration of treatment and the tissues irradiated. Generalised stomatitis may affect all soft tissues. Reduced salivary gland function, which causes xerostomia may take many months to return to normal function. People may need advice and support in coping with the symptoms.

Oral complications of radiotherapy to the head and neck include:

- Mucositis
- Xerostomia
- Loss of taste
- Radiation caries
- Hypersensitive teeth
- Periodontal disease
- Infections- particularly candidosis
- Osteoradionecrosis and osteomyelitis
- Trismus
- Dental defects.

Mucositis, characterised by red inflamed soft tissues that eventually slough off, is extremely painful and can affect the outcome of cancer therapy[6]. The most effective preventive approach is the frequent use of ice chips on the inflamed tissues to reduce sloughing[7].

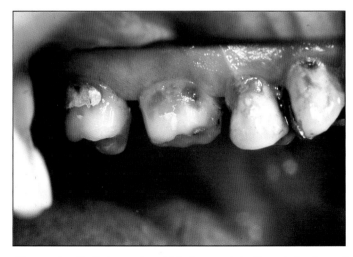

Figure 16.1 Radiation caries which characteristically encircles the necks of the teeth

Table 16.1 Nursing oral care guidelines

Prior to Cancer Therapy

Advise about Support groups: Cancer BACUP, Changing Faces, Let's Face It

	Objective	Nursing Action
1	Referral of all patients for a comprehensive assessment by a dentist prior to cancer therapy	Complete Oral Health Screening Chart and forward to dental team Liaise with dental team to develop and implement an individual care plan.
2	Advise on the oral side effects of treatment.	Provide written information on side effects of treatment.Give support and encouragement
3	Provide practical oral care	See Practical Oral Care (Table 16.2) Ensure oral hygiene equipment is available Give dietary advice in liaison with dietician Give support and encouragement with smoking cessation and alcohol problem

During Cancer Therapy

	Objective	Nursing Action
1	Maintenance of oral hygiene	Provide advice and assistance where appropriate. Follow Practical Oral Care (Table 16.2)
2	Inspection of the oral cavity should be carried out daily	Complete the Oral Assessment Guide daily and place in patient's individual care plan: contact dental team for guidance prior to completion if required Monitor any changes. Refer to dental team when indicated
3	Monitor compliance in performing oral care	Give support and encouragement Supervise and provide assistance; give instructions to carers where appropriate.
4	Pain control	Give topical / systemic analgesia as directed

During Cancer Therapy(cont)

	Objective	Nursing Action
5	Oral Candidal infection Thrush)	Give topical / systemic antifungal agents, as prescribed Stagger the use of chlorhexidine gluconate mouthwash and nystatin suspension by one hour
6	Manage xerostomia	Give advice to help with dry mouth Ensure recommended saliva substitute is prescribed and used where appropriate

After Cancer Therapy

	Objective	Nursing Action
1	Arrange follow-up visit to dental team	Provide patient or carer with contact telephone number Arrange an appointment Make an oral care entry in the summary notes / discharge letter to ensure follow up occurs after discharge
2	Reinforce preventive messages	Provide equipment for home care where appropriate Ensure patient information leaflet has been provided to support the advice given.

Reproduced with the kind permission of Professor June Nunn, Editor of Journal of Disability and Oral Health

Table 16.2 Practical Oral Care[1]

Care of the patient with natural teeth starts at Step 1. Care of the edentulous patient should start at Step 5.

	ORAL CARE	NOTES
1	Tooth brushing	Use a soft toothbrush and a Fluoride toothpaste. Encourage or assist with gentle thorough brushing of teeth and gums at least twice a day. If toothbrushing has to be discontinued, it should be resumed at the earliest opportunity.
2	Aqueous Chlorhexidine Gluconate Mouthwash	Use the mouthwash twice daily following toothbrushing. If toothbrushing is discontinued, use the mouthwash three to four times daily. N.B. Stagger the use of chlorhexidine mouthwash and nystatin antifungal agent - separate administration by at least one hour. Mouthwashes may need to be diluted for comfort eg 10ml mouthwash to 10ml water, ensuring the whole diluted volume is used
3	Fluoride mouthwash	Use a fluoride mouthwash daily as directed by the dental team. Fluoride gel may be used for children aged between three and six years as directed by the dental team. Use mouthwash during and after cancer therapy.
4	Dietary advice	Give preventive advice to reduce the risk of dental caries in liaison with a dietician. Place an emphasis on adequate hydration. Assist with healthy meal choices.
5	Gentle swabbing or oral tissues	Use polygon/gauze swabs soaked in chlorhexidine mouthwash to gently clean oral tissues. If the above cannot be tolerated, the swabs may be soaked in 0.9% saline (N.B. No antibacterial effect).
6	Moisten mouth and lips frequently	Advise regular sips of water. K.Y. jelly may be frequently applied to the lips, but should be removed when in the radiation field. Lubricate lips and tongue at night with flavourless salad oil. Use recommended artificial saliva substitutes.

7	Swabs for candidal infection	Take regular oral swabs for the detection of candida. Topical/systemic antifungal agents should be prescribed following the diagnosis of candida.
8	Care of dentures and obturators	Remove dentures and obturators after each meal and clean them thoroughly with a tooth or denture brush using unperfumed household soap. Clean over a basin of water to prevent damage if the appliance is dropped. Rinse well before replacing in cleaned mouth. Antifungal agents as prescribed may be applied to the fit surface of the denture prior to re-insertion. Remove dentures at night; clean and soak in an appropriate sodium hypo-chlorite cleanser (Milton, Dentural or Steradent if a metal denture is worn) for 30 minutes following removal; and store dry overnight. If dentures are to be left out for more than 24 hours, they should be stored damp. If dentures are stored away from the patient, they should be appropriately labelled. Advice on cleaning obturators will depend on the material the obturator is made from and will be given by the dental team
9	Denture and obturator wear	Leave dentures out of the mouth if there is any evidence of ulceration. Remove dentures at night. Moisten dentures with water or appropriate saliva substitute before replacing in mouth. Do not leave obturators out at night. If obturators cause ulceration, a specialist opinion should be sought.

Reproduced with the kind permission of Professor June Nunn, Editor of Journal of Disability and Oral Health

Symptoms of xerostomia include thick, ropey and viscous saliva; symptoms can develop shortly after radiotherapy. Xerostomia increases the risk of caries, periodontal disease, oral and salivary gland infections. Both xerostomia and damage to the taste buds contribute to loss of taste.

Dietary changes to cope with painful conditional requirements may increase the risk of caries, particularly if sugar rich food supplements are needed. This may be complicated by radiation caries (*Figure 16.1*). This has a typical presentation of cavities on the smooth surfaces encircling the crowns of the teeth at the gingival margins. Irradiation of developing teeth can result in defects to the teeth. Topical fluoride to prevent caries and chemical plaque control are essential.

Radiation damage to bone increases the risk of developing osteoradionecrosis and delaying healing. Section 16.8 provides the guidance necessary to plan treatment before, during and after cancer therapy.

16.7 Bone marrow transplantation

Bone marrow transplantation is a therapeutic technique that involves the replacement of dead cells in the bone marrow with live bone marrow cells, either from the same or from another individual.
Sources of bone marrow are:

- Allogeneic: healthy tissue from a compatible sibling
- Syngeneic: healthy tissue from an identical twin
- Autologous: tissue from the patient's own bone marrow.

Recent advances in treatment involve an initial course of chemotherapy, harvesting of bone marrow, then a subsequent higher dose which will eradicate the remaining cancer cells and bone marrow. This can then be followed by subsequent transplantation.

Graft versus Host Disease (GVHD) is a possible complication of Allogeneic transplant but advances in tissue typing are reducing the problem.

Chemotherapy and total body irradiation carried out before transplant are done in isolation, as the person is even more vulnerable to infection during this period. Some of the complications of bone marrow transplantation include:

- Poor nutrition
- Debilitation due to cytoxics

- Impaired healing
- Systemic bacterial infection
- Latent viral infections
- Impaired systemic defence
- Immunosuppression.

Oral complications of bone marrow transplantation are exacerbated by radiotherapy and chemotherapy.

16.8 Guidelines for the oral management of people requiring oncology therapy

The oral management of people in this group includes those undergoing:

- Radiotherapy
- Chemotherapy
- Bone marrow transplantation.

Recently published comprehensive guidelines include:

- Pathways of care
- Preventive and clinical programmes
- Tables describing oral complications
- Nursing oral care guidelines (*Table 16.1*)
- Comprehensive reference list underpinning all recommendations[8].
- Practical oral care (*Table 16.2*).

The pathway of care describes preventive and treatment interventions:

- Pre-treatment
- During cancer therapy
- Following cancer therapy.

Pre-treatment

Even though the time period between diagnosis and treatment may be short, as much of any outstanding urgent dental treatment and emergency care is carried out to allow time for healing. Early planning for any post treatment reconstruction should be undertaken. The planning for effective measures to maintain oral comfort during cancer therapy is required at this stage to minimise oral complications. The regimen should include:

- Full oral assessment including any dentures worn
- Dietary advice in liaison with the oncology team dietician as a high calorific diet may be needed during therapy
- Use of chlorhexidine mouthwash or gel before therapy
- Study models for later reconstruction if needed
- Temporary or permanent restorations if needed
- Adjustment of dentures if needed
- Undertaking any extractions up to three weeks prior to cancer therapy.

During cancer therapy

During cancer therapy it can expected that the person would experience some of the following oral changes:

- Mucositis
- Gingival bleeding
- Xerostomia
- Loss of taste
- Dysphagia.
- Changes in oral flora leading to:
- Oral candidiasis
- Acute periodontal disease
- Tooth sensitivity
- Dental pain
- Trismus.

The approaches during cancer therapy will require the close support of a dental hygienist to maintain as high a standard of oral hygiene as possible. The interventions required include:

- Frequent examinations of the mouth
- Toothbrushing and/or chlorhexidine mouthwash
- Fluoride drops/tablets or rinses
- Antifungals if oral candida detected
- Symptomatic relief of mucositis
- Saliva substitutes
- Lubrication of lips
- Cleaning of dentures with unperfumed soap\toothpaste and soaking in sodium hypochlorite

- Swabbing of the mouth with oral sponges if unable to use other cleaning techniques
- Avoiding foods and drinks that can cause discomfort including hard, hot, spicy foods, acidic drinks, tobacco and alcohol spirits
- Delaying elective dental treatment.

During the phase of cancer therapy it may be that the person will not be able to have regular contact with their primary care dentist due to their general condition. The role of the nursing team becomes increasingly important to assist with many of the above interventions. The nursing oral care guidelines are particularly important to guide the interventions (*Table 16.1*).

Following cancer therapy

There will be an increased risk of oral and dental disease following cancer therapy. This can last at least for 12 months and may lead to a permanent increased susceptibility. For children, there may have been damage to developing permanent teeth. If reconstructive surgery is required specialist support will be needed for care of obturators or implants. Some of the complications that can develop later include:

- Osteoradionecrosis following uncontrolled periodontal disease and/or dental extractions
- Gingival hyperplasia following cyclosporin
- Oral infections following immunosuppression
- Increased levels of dental caries including radiation caries
- Ongoing xerostomia

The basics of a good standard of oral hygiene and healthy diet will continue to be of high importance.

16.9 Summary

There is now a clear set of evidence based care pathways for the oral care of cancer patients. The challenge will be the maintaining of effective teamwork across all the disciplines involved. There is clear evidence that many of the oral complications of cancer therapy can be avoided or minimised by careful planning. This can enhance the person's comfort and well-being, improve the quality of life and reduce the risk of serious systemic infections.

References

1. BSDH Guidelines for the Oral Management of Oncology Patients Requiring Radiotherapy, Chemotherapy and Bone Marrow Transplantation. BSDH Working Group. *J Disabil Oral Health* 2001 **2**: 4.

2. Ibid

3. Clinical Guidelines. The Oral Management of Oncology Patients Requiring Radiotherapy:Chemotherapy:Bone Marrow Transplantation. The Dental Faculty of the Royal College of Surgeons of England.
   http://www.rcseng.ac.uk/dental/fds/clinical_guidelines/

4. Online National Statistics. http://www.statistics.gov.uk/

5. Aboutface facts. http://www.omfsaboutface.co.uk/index.htm

6. Caring for Cancer Patients. Patients Guide. Restorative Dentistry Oncology Clinic. http://www.rdoc.org.uk

7. Interventions for Preventing Oral Mucositis or Oral Candida in Patients with Cancer Receiving Chemotherapy (Excluding Neck Cancer). National Electronic Library for Health-Specialist Library-Oral Health (dentistry). http://www.nelh.nhs.uk

8. BSDH Guidelines for the Oral Management of Oncology Patients Requiring Radiotherapy, Chemotherapy and Bone Marrow Transplantation. BSDH Working Group. *J Disabil Oral Health* 2001 **2**: 3-14.

Chapter 17

People with mental health problems

17.1 Introduction

This chapter discusses the oral and dental problems that may occur in people with mental health problems. Brief accounts of diagnostic conditions are given to provide the reader with a reference point in relation to behaviour that may influence oral health.

17.2 Definitions

Mental illness is defined as clinically recognisable patterns of psychological symptoms causing acute or chronic ill health, personal distress or distress to others[1]. Mental illness is not a single 'condition'; people with a mental illness are not a homogenous group as mental illness describes a continuum ranging from minor distress to severe disorders of mind or behaviour[2]. Prevalence of 'mental illness' is comparable with cardiac and cardiovascular disorders as a major health problem in the UK.

The term mental illness is stigmatising and misleading since it implies a cut-off point between 'normal' behaviour and 'abnormal' behaviour or an 'abnormal' reaction to circumstances[3]. The borderline between 'mental health' and 'mental illness' is very fine and largely culturally defined. The term 'mental health problem' is a more acceptable way of describing the many conditions that cause mental and emotional distress as it recognises and acknowledges that many people experience mental distress and that a 'problem' is not necessarily an illness. It only becomes a serious problem when it interferes with the ability to cope with, or function on a day-to-day basis or when behaviour becomes a concern for others. Some people who experience severe or enduring mental health problems find diagnostic terminology unhelpful and prefer to talk about 'psychotic experiences'.

17.3 Prevalence of mental health problems

The entire population is susceptible to mental health problems so it is not a question of 'us and them'. At any one time, around one in six people of working age have a mental health problem[4]. Statistics compiled from a number of sources suggest that in the UK:

- 1 in 4 people will experience some kind of mental health problem each year
- 1 in 6 people will have depression some time in their life
- 1 in 10 people will have a 'disabling anxiety disorder' at some stage in their life

- 1 in 100 people will have a bipolar disorder or schizophrenia
- 20% of women and 14% of men have some form of mental illness
- 18% of women experience a 'neurotic' disorder compared with 11% of men
- Men are three times more likely to have alcohol dependence and twice as likely to be drug dependent[3].

In pre-school children:

- 15% will have a mild mental health problem
- 7% will have a severe mental health problem[3].

In adolescents:

- 6% of boys and 16% of girls aged 16-19 are thought to have some form of mental health problem
- 10-20% of young people involved in criminal activity are thought to have a 'psychiatric disorder'[3].

In older people:

- 15% of people over 65 have depression
- 5% over 65 and 10-20% over 80 have dementia[3].

So the lay concept of 'mental illness' as being a condition that affects 'other' people must be challenged. Estimates are based upon diagnosis through contact with general medical services and are probably an underestimate of the true prevalence.

17.4 Classification of mental health problems

As discussed in the introduction to this section, the definitions used will focus on medical diagnostic terminology. Mental health problems are categorised in different ways:

- Organic disorders are a direct result of brain malfunction
  e.g. delirium caused by trauma or Alzheimer's disease
- Functional disorders are not caused by simple structural abnormalities of the brain.

Organic causes such as recognisable organic brain disease, affect relatively few people except in older age groups. In certain conditions, heredity may be a contributory factor whereas in Huntington's disease, heredity is a known factor (Chapter 13). The high incidence of Alzheimer's disease in people with Down syndrome may be related to premature ageing and/or genetic factors. However, most mental health problems are classed as functional.

Diagnostic categories can also be subdivided in to neuroses and psychoses, although some conditions such as 'personality disorders' fall outside these categories[3].

Neuroses are regarded as severe forms of normal experience. They include stress-related and somatoform disorders e.g. anxiety disorders, phobias, depression and obsessive-compulsive disorders (OCD).

Psychoses are more severe and involve a distortion of the individual's perception of reality. Psychoses are often accompanied by delusions and/or hallucinations. The commonest psychotic disorders are schizophrenia, bi-polar disorders (manic depression) and psychotic depression. The WHO ICD Classification of Diseases (1993) also provides an international classification of mental and behavioural disorders[1].

Behaviour associated with alcohol or substance abuse may have a psychiatric component. The effects of major trauma or severe life-threatening conditions may lead to a range of individual emotional reactions. Biochemical factors associated with endocrinal changes are suggested causes of post-natal or menopausal depression, although environmental factors cannot be excluded. Physical illness and biochemical deficiencies are also quoted as possible factors.

Stress, family or social pressures, poor or inadequate housing, and homelessness are contributory factors. More than half the homeless in London are in touch with specialist mental health services[5]. Females are generally more often admitted to hospital, especially for depression. Some disorders appear to have a higher incidence in certain racial groups; while the prevalence of schizophrenia appears to be higher in social classes IV and V, although the stigma attached to the condition and subsequent downward drift may account for the reported class distribution.

Pressure to achieve has lead to an increased value attached to success, autonomy and self-reliance. Stress is increasingly accepted as an aetiological factor in the development of mental health problems. An isolated and relatively insignificant event in the context of other factors may be the precipitating factor.

Historical patterns of custodial care in large psychiatric institutions are gradually changing. The closure of large institutions and provision of care at home or in sheltered or supported housing and day centres reflects the changing patterns of treatment for people with mental health problems. However, the effects of long-term institutionalisation, which may lead to deterioration in motivation and personal care, will be increasingly evident in the community as hospitals close and financial support for community care is under pressure.

17.5 Oral health and disease

With advances in treatment, particularly the development of medication that controls or reduces symptoms, there is evidence to suggest that individuals on long-term psychiatric medication are more at risk of oral disease. Depending on the diagnosis, medication may often have to be taken for life. Studies report dental neglect in adults with chronic mental health problems in a range of settings; oral disease is associated with mood, motivation, life-style, and problems of compliance with regular dental attendance[6-14]. The primary factor is considered to be the mental disorder, while associated factors are financial constraints, life-style, poor oral hygiene and the xerostomic side-effects of long-term psychotropic medication.

Dry mouth was a consistent feature of a group with mental illness compared with the control[13]. Dental caries of the smooth surfaces and root surfaces (mainly seen in older people) was higher in the sample with mental illness, possibly due to reported increased consumption of carbonated drinks (*Figure 1.7, 1.8*). Periodontal disease was also more severe.

Side-effects of many of the major psychiatric drugs are highlighted in the literature and summarised in *Table 17.1*. The side-effects of long-term psychotropic medication in reducing salivary secretions are an important risk factor for dental decay (caries), periodontal disease and oral infections. Poor compliance with anti-psychotic medication justifies the use of sustained-release medication, which can be administered orally or by injection at prescribed intervals. Advances in psychiatric medication have had a significant impact on the treatment and prognosis of mental illness but prescription of long-term medication without advising the individual of the range of possible side-effects is not acceptable. There does not appear to be any documentary evidence to demonstrate that information on side-effects is routinely provided; information should include advice on oral side-effects, the implications for oral health, and appropriate counselling from health professionals.

The side-effects of major psychiatric drugs may be relatively unimportant compared to the potential for relief of symptoms. However, the oral side-effects of medication on oral and dental disease need to be highlighted.

Table 17.1 Oral and facial side-effects of antipsychotic medication

Drug	Possible oral side-effects
Antidepressants	
Tricyclic antidepressants	Dry mouth
	Involuntary facial
	movements
Monoamine oxidase inhibitors	Dry mouth
SSRIs (selective serotonin re-uptake inhibitors)	Dry mouth
Hypnotics	
Promethazine hydrochloride	Dry mouth
Anxiolytics	
Diazepam	Salivation changes
Alprazolam	Salivation changes
Clorazepate dipotassium	Salivation changes
Lorazepam	Salivation changes
Oxazepam	Salivation changes
Hydroxyzine hydrochloride	Dry mouth
Anti-psychotic drugs	
Phenothiazines	Tardive dyskinesia *
	Dry mouth
Butyrophenones	Tardive dyskinesia *
	Dry mouth
Anti-manic drugs	
Carbamazepine	Erythema multiforme
	(Stevens-Johnson syndrome)
	Involuntary facial
	movements
Anti-parkinsonian drugs	Dry mouth

Source: Dental Practitioners' Formulary. 2002-2004.
(* Tardive dyskinesia – involuntary facial movements)

Attention to oral hygiene, prevention and diet is essential, together with regular dental attendance to advise, monitor and treat, if oral side-effects are to be minimised. This chapter will concentrate on the commoner conditions and their potential for oral disease.

17.6 Barriers to oral health

Illness often leads to a deterioration in self-care. Important factors include a lack of motivation and a temporary or permanent loss of ability, knowledge and skill. Oral care may already have a low priority, and in periods of severe mental impairment, oral hygiene may have an even lower priority or be non-existent. Traditional barriers to dental care which apply to the total population will also apply to the non-homogeneous proportion who experience mental health problems. Socio-economic factors, life-style, personality changes and psychological factors which affect 'normal function' may interfere with relationships. Mood changes, behaviour or inability to function 'normally' may act as additional barriers to self-care and to seeking help and treatment, including dental treatment (*Table 17.2*).

Table 17.2 Behavioural factors in mental illness

Impaired ability to learn	Anxiety
Deterioration in personal care	Fear
Poor motivation	Delusions
Amnesia	Hallucinations
Disorientation	Paranoia
Mood changes	

Guidelines published by the British Society for Disability and Oral Health (BSDH, 2000) provide a comprehensive summary of factors that influence oral health for this client group:

- Type, severity and stage of mental illness
- Client's mood motivation and self-esteem
- Lack of personal perception of oral health problems
- Client's habits, lifestyle and ability to sustain self-care and dental attendance
- Environmental factors which mitigate against preservation of self-care
- Socio-economic factors which limit choices for healthy living
- Language and culture
- Lack of guidance on how to access information or dental services
- Oral side-effects of medication in particular the impact of xerostomia

- Attitudes to oral care and knowledge of health professionals and health care workers
- Dental team's attitude to, and knowledge of, mental health problems
- Local dental personnel unable or unwilling to provide adequate dental care[15].

The reader is advised to access this report, which is available on the Society's website[15].

17.7 Side-effects of medication

Most of the major drugs used to alleviate or control psychiatric symptoms have side-effects. The most commonly used medications are:

- Tranquillisers
- Long-acting tranquillisers
- Tricyclic antidepressants
- Monoamine oxidase inhibitors (MAOIs)
- Selective serotonin uptake inhibitors (SSRIs)
- Hypnotics
- Anti-psychotic drugs
- Lithium and its derivatives
- Anti-parkinsonian drugs.

Side-effects may be physiological and produce other behavioural symptoms or mood changes. Oral side-effects are summarised in Chapter 8, although many drugs also cause blood dyscrasias which may be reflected in the soft tissues of the mouth.

The most common oral side-effect of psychiatric medication is dry mouth (xerostomia) caused by reduced salivary secretion. The implications of dry mouth as a factor in increasing the risks of dental caries, periodontal disease and oral infections are covered in Chapter 2. Signs, symptoms, and the treatment of dry mouth are summarised in *Table 17.3*. Other side-effects which affect mood may influence oral care. Involuntary facial movements make dental treatment difficult for patient and clinician; anti-parkinsonian drugs may be prescribed to counter involuntary movements such as tardive dyskinesia.

Table 17.3 Dry mouth (xerostomia)

Signs and symptoms		Management
Dry mouth		Improve oral hygiene
Difficulty with:	speech	Avoid sugar based drinks
	swallowing	(dentate)
	dentures	Frequent sips of iced water
Disturbed taste sensation		Suck chips of ice
Increased rate of caries		Saliva substitutes
Increased periodontal disease		Chlorhexidine mouthwash, gel
Oral & salivary gland infections		or spray
		Evian atomised water spray
		Refer to dentist or doctor
		for advice

17.8 Neuroses

Neuroses are disorders of emotional or intellectual functioning which do not deprive the individual of contact with reality. These include conditions such as:

- Anxiety and phobic states
- Hysterical states
- Obsessive-compulsive disorders (OCD)
- Post-Traumatic Stress Disorder (PTSD)
- Grief and neurotic depression.

Anxiety and phobia

Anxiety states are common; 1 in 10 people are likely to have a 'disabling anxiety disorder' at some point in their life[3]. Fear and anxiety, often amounting to panic, characterise this unwelcome state. Among the classic features of 'flight and fight', caused by the action of the sympathetic autonomic nervous system, are the common symptoms of increased anxiety, hypertension, alertness, loss of appetite and dry mouth.

Dentists are familiar with anxiety as a daily feature of dental practice. It is often a learnt response from parents and family or due to previous unpleasant or traumatic dental experiences. Fear and anxiety about dental treatment has a direct influence on the attendance patterns of people who mainly seek dental care for relief of pain. About a third of adults with natural teeth agreed that they always feel anxious about going to the dentist.[16] Dental fear and anxiety are more marked among subjects with high levels of general fearfulness[17].

Non-attendance leads to lack of/or delayed treatment. Without resorting to treatment under a general anaesthetic or intravenous sedation, completely pain-free dental treatment may be impossible, thus reinforcing and justifying the original fear. Tooth loss may be inevitable. Hostile behaviour can mask the patient's fear and create a communication barrier between patient and clinician that reinforces the phobia.

Specific phobias that interfere with 'normal' daily living act as barriers to dental care. Needle phobics need support in obtaining appropriate treatment to enable them to overcome this problem. Increasingly, desensitisation, relaxation techniques and hypnosis are being used to help patients with needle phobia receive dental treatment. Agoraphobia and claustrophobia are common phobic disorders. Agoraphobics confined to their own home are isolated from information and services. There is clearly a need for local information on available domiciliary dental services to be made known to this group, carers and mental health professionals. This could be achieved by an out-reach approach to professional and voluntary agencies involved in identifying and supporting people with mental health problems.

Hysterical neuroses

There are no demonstrable oral problems associated with hysterical states, although a number of physical complaints without a demonstrable organic cause have been reported. These may affect the oral cavity and include:

- Pain
- Anaesthesia
- Delusional halitosis
- Dysphagia
- Cancerophobia.

Oral symptoms may be the first manifestation of a mental health problem; a third of patients attending a temperomandibular dysfuntion joint clinic had evidence of a mental disorder[18]. In Munchausen syndrome, patients may fabricate histories and symptoms for the sake of on undergoing repeated operations; Munchausen syndrome-by-proxy describes a parent or carer who fabricates symptoms and demands medical or surgical treatment for a child[19]. It is important that oral complaints are fully investigated by referral for a dental opinion. This provides the opportunity to eliminate oral or systemic disease, and provide reassurance where necessary or facilitate referral to psychiatric or psychological services.

Obsessive compulsive disorders

These are rarely centred on the mouth but may include compulsive tooth brushing, the excessive use of mouthwashes or obsession with the possibility of oral infection, including cancer. If there is an obsession with maintaining oral hygiene, rigorous oral care using incorrect or over-vigorous tooth brushing techniques may lead to enamel abrasion and recession of the gingival margins. Dental advice or treatment may be sought repeatedly as a means of reinforcing or confirming an obsession, and referral for psychiatric assessment may be initiated by the dentist.

Depressive neuroses

Reactive or neurotic depression, which is characterised by mental withdrawal and a lowered mood, may be an over-reaction to 'normal' loss as in grief, or as a response to physical illness or a major change in life circumstances. Neurotic depressive illness occurs most often in young adults as a reaction to stress.

General apathy, loss of appetite and sleep disturbances, together with periods of anxiety or agitation, may lead to deterioration in self-care. Depression may also be associated with a number of orofacial complaints:

- Atypical facial pain
- Burning mouth or sore tongue
- Pain and dysfunction of the temporomandibular joint
- Oral delusions: abnormal discharges
- Dry mouth
- Spots or lumps
- Halitosis
- Disturbances of taste sensation[19].

Some of the above may be directly attributed to the side-effects of medication. MAO inhibitors and tricyclics are common treatments for depression; side-effects include dry mouth. This is particularly notable in tricyclics which have a strong anticholinergic effect, but is reported to be less of a problem with the newer tricyclic drugs. Dry mouth may have a psychological component; a dental opinion should be sought to eliminate oral pathology, establish an oral health promotion programme to alleviate the symptoms and referral to mental health services if a psychogenic cause is suspected.

Temporomandibular joint (TMJ) pain may be associated with compulsive or stress-related habits, such as clenching, chewing or grinding (bruxism). Loss of molar teeth is a common contributory factor; provision of dentures to replace missing teeth and restore the occlusion may produce relief. Soft splints or bite-guards that cover occlusal surfaces may provide relief and prevent recurrence. Analgesics, muscle relaxants and mild anxiolytics may be prescribed for pain relief.

17.9 Psychoses

The term psychosis is used to describe the distortion of a person's perception of reality. Psychoses are characterised by a profound and essential disturbance in the individual's appreciation of the nature of their environment and their response to it, and although a lack of insight into the conditions is regarded as a characteristic of psychosis, individuals vary in their ability to perceive their mental state of mind. Psychosis is often accompanied by delusions involving a strong belief held on false or insufficient grounds and / or hallucinations that can involve any of the five senses. Paranoia, a persecutory delusion may also be a feature. Psychosis is a symptom of some of the more serious forms of mental health problems such as:

- Affective disorders: Psychotic depression
  Bipolar disorders (manic depression)
- Organic cerebral disorders: Delirium
  Epilepsy (Chapter 13)
  Dementia
- Schizophrenia
- Disorders of old age
- Puerperal psychosis
- Substance abuse

and some forms of personality disorder. Alcohol, infections and brain disease can also result in psychotic episodes.

Psychotic depression

This is considered to be a pathological condition characterised by acute misery, malaise and despair that grossly exceed a 'normal' response to the precipitating loss or crisis. In some cases it occurs spontaneously; the individual has a distorted view of reality, and possibly delusions and / or hallucinations. Involutional melancholia describes depressive illness in the 45-65 age group; in women, this is accompanied by agitation and may be associated with the menopause.

Familial tendencies, stress, neurochemistry and the effects of debilitating physical illness, particularly endocrine disorders, are considered to be aetiological factors. Psychotic depression occurs commonly as a secondary feature of other psychiatric conditions, such as schizophrenia, anxiety states and alcoholism. Cognitive theories view psychotic depression as a syndrome of aggression turned inwardly against the self.

Mood changes, generalised withdrawal, apathy and inertia, agitation, anxiety, fatigue and physiological disturbances in sleep, appetite and digestion have an inevitable effect on self-care. Oral care may have no importance in such a distressing and gloomy, even suicidal, state of mind. Treatment is with a combination of antidepressants and symptomatic drugs, together with supportive psychotherapy and electroconvulsive therapy (ECT). The major drugs used for the treatment of psychotic depression are:

- Tricyclic antidepressants
- Tetracyclic antidepressants
- Bicyclic antidepressants
- Monoamine oxidase inhibitors (MAOIs)
- Combination drugs (*Table 17.1*).

Tardive dyskinesia is unlikely to occur with the small doses of major tranquillisers found in combination drugs. Some antipsychotic drugs with antidepressant properties, e.g. flupenthixol, tryptophan and fluvoxamine, are reported to have fewer side-effects and are less likely to reduce salivary secretion. ECT is carried out under general anaesthesia therefore a pre-anaesthetic dental assessment may be advisable to identify mobile teeth and loose crowns or bridges on teeth that might be displaced during intubation.

Bipolar disorders (manic depression)

Manic psychoses are often referred to as bipolar disorders; they are characterised by periods of extreme elation and irritability and frequently associated with depressive episodes. During the manic phase, task-orientated attention is lacking, while during the depressive phase, motivation and drive are absent. Bipolar disorders are reported to first occur in young adults, whereas in the elderly they may indicate organic disease or be secondary to the effect of drugs.

Prognosis for treatment of the manic phase has dramatically improved with the use of lithium. Anti-depressive medication may be prescribed during the depressive phase. Lithium interacts with a number of other drugs; interaction with clozapine, haloperidol, phenothiazines and sulpiride increase the risk of extra-pyramidal symptoms such as tardive dyskinesia. This is a distressing symptom and poses management problems for dental treatment. Lithium may precipitate cardiac arrhythmias, which pose a risk for general anaesthesia; it is recommended that lithium is stopped 24 hours before major surgery involving general anaesthesia. Preventive oral hygiene to avoid the need for a dental general anaesthetic is important.

One of the few studies of oral health in bipolar disorders reports that during the depressive phase, most subjects with natural teeth had severe gingivitis and a total disregard for oral hygiene[20]. Three subjects reported generalised stomatitis when lithium therapy was recommended, while 78% of the sample reported dry mouth and a few reported a burning sensation in the lips and tongue, difficulty with speech, and changes in taste sensation. The subjects' response to dry mouth (xerostomia) was mostly an increased consumption of 'candy' and drinks with a high sugar content to relieve thirst – behaviour that predisposes to dental caries. However, during the manic phase, dry mouth was not a problem. The sample in the manic phase was too small to draw conclusive comparisons but the authors concluded that their dental condition appeared to be a function of their emotional state and its influence on both salivary flow and poor oral hygiene. In those individuals who increased their intake of cariogenic food and drink, the potential for oral and dental disease was greater.

Further research is needed to identify the relevant importance of attention, motivation and drive in the manic and depressive phases, changes in salivary flow during the depressive phases, and the oral side-effects of medication. Dietary counselling and advice on improving oral hygiene should be a priority, as well as advice on management of a dry mouth and the use of saliva substitutes. Changes in life-style may be more difficult to achieve but regular dental attendance should be encouraged.

Organic cerebral disorders

Organic brain disease may underlie physical symptoms of delirium, epilepsy and dementia.

Delirium: Delirium, sometimes known as 'acute organic disorder' or 'acute confusional state' is more common than dementia. It is characterised by an altered state of consciousness, distraction, disorientation in time and place, poor concentration, attention and memory and slow or muddled thinking. The main causes are physical illness and drug reactions. If the underlying cause is treated, symptoms resolve. Personal care including oral hygiene is likely to be poor during illness. Disturbed behaviour may be controlled with chlorpromazine, haloperidol or thioridazine, all of which reduce salivary secretions.

Dementia: Dementia is defined as 'organic loss of intellectual functioning' and is the result of deterioration in previously normal brain function. It is global in that it affects all faculties in a previously alert individual, and is generally considered to be irreversible. Onset occurs primarily in later life. Dementia affects 5% of people over the age of 65 and 10-20% over 80[3]. Approximately 18,500 people with dementia are under the age of 65[21]. There are over a hundred different types of dementia; the most common are Alzheimer's disease, cerebro-vascular dementia and Lewy Body dementia. Dementia can also occur in association with Parkinson's disease. Head injury, raised intra-cranial pressure, brain tumours, alcohol or hypothyroidism are less common causes that are more amenable to treatment (*Table 17.4*).

Table 17.4 Aetiological factors in dementia

Type of dementia	Aetiology
Primary degenerative brain disease	Alzheimer's disease
	Pick's disease
	Lewy Body dementia
	Huntington's disease
	Creutzfeld-Jakob disease
	AIDS related dementia
Cerebrovascular disease	Atherosclerotic dementia (multi-infarct dementia)
Dementia secondary to other conditions	Brain injury
	Anoxic brain damage
	Infection
	Poisoning
	Metabolic and endocrine disorders
	Neoplasms
	Hydrocephalus
	Epilepsy

Alzheimer's disease (AD) also called pre-senile and senile dementia is the most common form of dementia. Necrotic areas of the cerebral cortex were first described by Alzheimer in 1906. The identification of biochemical brain changes, in particular a decrease in the level of acetylcholine transferase, have prompted research into new drug treatments. The first sign is often an exaggerated loss of memory for recent events, which progresses with confusion, loss of language function and memory failure due to dementia. Behavioural problems and severe dementia develop in the later stages. The course of the disease is variable and may be aggravated by isolation, sensory deprivation, physical illness, the side-effects of medication, and by family pressures and tensions.

Genetic factors are increasingly recognised as playing a role in some forms of AD, although other factors are involved. Specific genetic defects have been identified in chromosome 21 (the abnormal chromosome in Down syndrome), which is involved in the formation of excessive amounts of protein found in the brains of Alzheimer's subjects. In the rare familial form, autsomal-dominant inheritance has been identified.

Alzheimer's disease is irreversible. Recent drug treatments, which act by inhibiting acetylcholinesterase, may slow down the rate of deterioration in mild to moderate dementia. Memantine, a new drug licensed for middle to late stages of AD is currently under consideration by the National Institute for Clinical Excellence. Anti-psychotic medication may be prescribed to control agitation. Oral side effects of new medication should be noted and reported.

Lewy Body dementia is the second most frequent cause of dementia in older adults, although younger people can be affected[22]. It is a neuro-degenerative disorder associated with abnormal brain structures (Lewy bodies). It is not yet understood whether this is a distinct condition or perhaps a variant of Alzheimer's disease or Parkinson's disease (Chapter 13). Symptoms can range from traditional parkinsonian effects to those of Alzheimer's disease. Visual hallucination may be one of the first symptoms. Treatment is symptomatic but antiparkinsonian medication may worsen symptoms such as delusion and hallucination. Atypical antispsychotic medications are more successful.

Pre-senile dementia refers to dementia occurring before the age of 65. It includes early onset AD, Pick's disease, Huntington's disease, Creutzfeldt-Jakob disease (CJD) and AIDS related dementia. Pick's disease is a rare inherited degenerative condition that affects the frontal and parietal lobes; it occurs between the ages of 45 to 65, has a slow course with socially inappropriate or uninhibited behaviour. CJD is a very rare cause of pre-senile dementia; it is characterised by progressive dementia and sometimes muscle wasting, tremor, athetosis and spastic dysarthria (Chapter 15). Huntington's disease (HD) is well known as a hereditary cause that occurs mainly in middle age (Chapter 13). A minority of people who are HIV positive develop dementia; this is thought to be caused by direct damage of brain cells by human immunodeficiency virus (HIV) (Chapter 15). The prevalence of Alzheimer's type dementia in Down syndrome is more than double that of the general population. Sexually transmitted diseases are on the increase therefore dementia as a result of untreated syphilis must be considered. Deep ulcers affecting the skin and oral tissues, which may progress to destroy underlying bone are a feature of neurosyphilis. The most significant oral symptom is leukoplakia (*Figure 15.3*), a condition characterised by thick white patches, which occur particularly on the surface of the tongue. These lesions have a high potential for malignant change. Syphilitic cardiovascular disease may affect the management of dental treatment.

Atherosclerotic dementia: This is generally referred to as multi-infarct dementia and is caused by cerebro-vascular disease. Multiple small haemorrhages and infarcts caused by atherosclerosis of the cranial arteries result in localised areas of brain damage. Depression, mood swings and a tendency to weep, are more typical of this type of dementia. Antidepressants prescribed for depression may reduce salivary flow.

Oral problems in dementia

Higher levels of caries and periodontal disease and poor oral hygiene are reported in subjects with dementia[23-25]. Memory loss, confusion and impaired ability to perform perceptuo-motor skills, lead to neglect and deterioration in personal care. Oral health will be affected, and personal and oral care will in most cases become the responsibility of a carer.

The individual's ability to cooperate for treatment or adjust to new dentures decreases with their ability to cooperate. Side-effects of anticonvulsant therapy must be considered. The risk of oral disease is increased by the use of anticholinergics to treat depression, involuntary movements and other medical conditions; other medication may also reduce salivary flow. Information and advice on oral care and dental attendance to prevent oral disease and provide treatment before the ability to cooperate deteriorates should be available to carers in the early stages of disease.

The burden of responsibility and care rests mainly with family and relatives who suffer considerable personal and emotional hardship, caring for a relative whose condition is inevitably going to deteriorate, and in many cases with insufficient support from statutory services. Most carers indicated that dental care was important, and more than half reported that the person cared for had dental problems in the previous year[26]. The inability to ascertain whether a person with dementia is in pain can be distressing. The dental profession's lack of awareness of the problems associated with dementia suggest the need for greater interdisciplinary training and co-operation.

Dental care provided in the unfamiliar surroundings of a dental surgery may be disorientating for a person with dementia. This may be reduced by being in the familiar surroundings of the home environment. Domiciliary dental care offers an alternative but is less popular except for older dependent people who are edentulous[26]. This may be due to carers' lack of knowledge of portable dental equipment and the range of treatments that can be provided at home. Regrettably, domiciliary dental care is not universally available but the situation may change as the public becomes more aware of the requirements of the Disability Discrimination Act (1995)[27].

The underlying cause of dementia, the effects of mental decline, medication and deteriorating personal care on the individual's oral health must be considered. It is important that carers are made aware of the predominant oral infections that occur and the techniques for managing oral care in a sensible, safe and practical way. Health professionals have an important role in counselling and informing carers of risks to oral health, providing preventive advice and facilitating contact with a suitable and sympathetic source of dental care. Guidelines for the oral health care of people with dementia will be published in the near future.

Schizophrenia

Historically, schizophrenia was thought to be an expression of 'split personality', epitomising the concept of 'madness' – a view which is still promoted by much of the tabloid press, and sensationalised by ignorance and misuse of the term. Originally called 'dementia praecox', schizophrenia is now accepted as the term for a group of severe emotional disorders, which are characterised by a progressive disintegration of the individual's personality and a psychological detachment from the real world. Symptoms include misinterpretation and retreat from reality, delusions, hallucinations, indifference, inappropriate moods, withdrawn and sometimes bizarre or regressive behaviour. Schizophrenia is being rejected as a medical diagnosis by some people diagnosed with schizophrenia and some professional and non-professional carers but there is certain agreement that help and support is needed for those affected.

Schizophrenia is the most common psychosis. It is estimated that 1 in 100 people will experience one episode, and two-thirds will go on to have further episodes. Approximately 3% of the population have a schizophrenic personality, which is characterised by social and personal withdrawal, sometimes with eccentricity, shyness and reticence, hypersensitivity and suspicious tendencies. The exact cause of schizophrenia is unknown but it has been established beyond doubt that schizophrenia is a biological disorder although environmental factors have a critical role in the aetiology of schizophrenia. There is a familial link, which is thought to be genetic in origin. Research into brain structure and function in schizophrenia is in its infancy but physical and bio-chemical theories are emerging. In some cases, street drugs (ecstasy, LSD, amphetamines, cannabis) are triggers.

Onset is usually in early adulthood and generally appears about 10 years earlier in males than in females. Differences occur in the acute and chronic phases of schizophrenia. In the acute phase, symptoms may include hallucinations, delusions and thought disorder and in the chronic phase, flattening of emotion, social withdrawal and reduced verbal communication. No two cases are identical and the reader is advised to consult other sources for a greater understanding of this complex condition that leads to mental impairment.

Drugs which control hallucinations, reduce severe thought disorders and delusions; they have a calming effect and have dramatically changed the outcome for many people diagnosed with schizophrenia. Behaviour becomes less anti-social, thus facilitating better integration into society. A significant feature of this illness is that the individual may have little insight into their illness and therefore compliance with regular anti-psychotic medication may be poor. Medication is usually taken for life; long-acting depot preparations given orally or by injection help to overcome non-compliance. Drugs commonly used include phenothiazines and butyrophenones. The tranquillising effect is considered of secondary importance to the effective control of delusional symptoms. Many side-effects are reported which include dry mouth and tardive dyskinesia (involuntary facial and bodily movements); the latter may be irreversible. Parkinsonian side-effects include:

- Mask-like facial appearance due to stiff and weak musculature
- Hand tremor
- Pill-rolling movements of the fingers
- Restlessness
- Forward and shuffling gait.

Side-effects vary depending on the specific drug prescribed, dose, duration, and individual susceptibility. Haloperidol is reported to have less effect on salivary secretions; however other side-effects described above are more common. There are no specific oral and dental problems related to schizophrenia. However, oral delusions such as teeth being 'bugged' or fitted with 'transmitters' have been encountered by the authors in some in-patients. In one case, six anterior crowns were very neatly removed by the patient using a pair of electrical pliers; it was difficult to convince the patient that the temporary crowns fitted as a replacement had not been 'tampered with'.

Management of dental treatment may be more difficult in the acute phase and if tardive dyskinesia or Parkinsonian features are present. While the management of schizophrenic symptoms must be the priority, every effort should be made to encourage good oral care and dietary control of sugars to reduce the oral health risks of a dry mouth.

Psychosis in older people

Almost all psychiatric disorders increase with age and peak in old age. Some disorders represent the chronic state of earlier diagnosed disease. The most characteristic are:

- Delusional states
- Depression
- Dementia of organic origin
- Paraphrenia (schizophrenia of late onset)
- Neurotic symptoms
- Personality deterioration.

The causes have largely been covered in earlier sections of this chapter. Severe depressive reactions may occur as a consequence of ageing and loss, such as bereavement, loneliness, progressive illness and an impoverishment in quality of life. Loss of memory, sensory impairment, lack of social contact and social isolation contribute to paranoid states. Physical illness may be associated with delusions. A diagnosis of paraphrenia is only made when there is evidence of personality deterioration. Deterioration in oral hygiene skills, ability to cooperate for treatment and the oral side-effects of medication must be considered.

17.10 Psychosomatic disorders

In viewing health and illness holistically, it is evident that some illnesses will be psychogenic in origin. The complex interaction of the various anatomical, physiological and biochemical systems is still poorly understood. Emotional responses which are a combination of biophysical changes and external experience, can lead an individual to believe that they are suffering from an imaginary pain or illness, which is subjectively real.

It is beyond the scope of this book to explore this interesting subject in depth, but if an oral complaint is expressed, then a dental opinion should be obtained to eliminate oral pathology. Burning mouth, dry mouth, halitosis, disturbed taste sensations and oral or facial pain are common psychogenic complaints. Interdisciplinary assessment may be necessary to reach a diagnosis.

17.11 Anorexia and bulimia

Eating disorders develop as outward signs of inner emotional or psychological distress or problems. Anorexia nervosa and bulimia nervosa receive the greatest attention because they are potentially life threatening but binge eating disorders are probably more common. Eating disorders are reported to affect mainly young females who have an obsession or phobia with weight gain and body image. However these conditions are reported to be increasing in young males in Western society. The incidence increased fourfold from the mid-sixties to the late seventies and early eighties in a climate of heightened cultural pressure to conform to a stereotypical image of being slim.

Anorexia nervosa is characterised by a misperception of body image. Individuals with anorexia nervosa believe they are overweight even when they are grossly underweight. The incidence is 7 per 100,000 and the prevalence ranges from 0.1 to 1% of young females[28]. Approximately 4,000 new cases are identified annually in the UK. The individual has a profound aversion to food, which in extreme cases leads to starvation.

Bulimia nervosa is characterised by over-eating, sometimes accompanied by self-induced vomiting. It is more common than anorexia nervosa. The incidence ranges from 8.6 to 14 per 100,000 of the population[28]. Between 1-2% of adolescent girls and young women are affected. Anorexics are generally below body weight for their age and height whereas bulimics can be overweight. Bulimia is thought to be stress related and bingeing often includes a high proportion of cariogenic food. Laxatives are sometimes taken to induce weight loss. Both conditions can co-exist or alternate in the same individual and may be regarded as a hysterical condition.

The objectives of treatment are to establish rapport, followed by nursing, dietary and supportive regimes to restore body weight, with therapy to deal with the underlying psychopathological symptoms. Malnutrition, dehydration, symptomatic behaviour and drugs used in the treatment of anxiety or vomiting may affect the mouth; oral symptoms are summarised in *Table 17.5*. Anaemia may be secondary to malnutrition and poses a risk for increased susceptibility to oral infections and for treatment under general anaesthesia.

Table 17.5 Oral symptoms in eating disorders

Tooth erosion secondary to vomiting, reflux and regurgitation (Figure 2.3)

Possible changes in salivary secretion

Soft tissue lesions: angular cheilitis, glossitis, ulceration (self-inflicted or due to trauma)

Enlargement of parotid salivary glands

Anaemia[29]

Immediate and excessive toothbrushing after vomiting may account for excessive wear of tooth enamel. Ulcers in the pharynx due to accidental trauma to induce vomiting are also reported. Some anti-emetics to reduce vomiting also reduce salivary secretion.

Dentists are likely to encounter patients with undiagnosed eating disorders. A dentist may be the first to make a provisional diagnosis of an eating disorder, particularly when a thin young female presents with erosion of the palatal and lingual surfaces[29]. Preventive advice and treatment for the oral effects include:

- Fluoride toothpaste
- Fluoride mouthwash or gel
- Topical fluoride professionally applied
- Splints to protect teeth during vomiting.

Professional treatment will be required for angular cheilitis and oral trauma.

17.12 Alcohol and substance abuse

Substance use, abuse and dependence are increasing. The high incidence of HIV amongst intravenous drug users has raised the profile of substance abuse in health promotion targets. Psychiatric illness is reported in both alcoholism and in the illicit use of drugs. Personal neglect may also be a feature.

Blackouts, hallucinations, delirium tremens following withdrawal, Korsakoff's syndrome and alcoholic dementia summarise the mental health problems associated with alcohol abuse. Oral problems in alcoholism are frequently related to neglect and poor oral hygiene; they include:

- Advanced dental caries
- Periodontal disease
- Angular cheilitis
- Oral signs of anaemia.

Other problems arise due to accidental maxillofacial injury and trauma. Medical conditions associated with alcohol abuse may affect general health and seriously influence suitability for treatment under general anaesthesia. The incidence of oral cancer in alcohol and substance users is discussed in Chapters 1 and 2.

Addiction to narcotics and other substances is a complex subject. Mental health problems may be related to addiction or withdrawal, or of the use of hallucinogenic drugs. High levels of dental caries are reported in drug addicts[12]. Xerostomia, 'fiery red gingivitis', white patches, papilloma, candidosis, and oral and pharyngeal carcinoma are reported in cannabis smokers[30]. Dental caries and periodontal disease are increased in cocaine addiction. Solvent abuse, which mainly occurs in the early teens, may lead to paranoid or aggressive outbursts; the practice of glue sniffing can cause lesions around the mouth.

Dental treatment may be more difficult to provide due to withdrawal or behavioural changes, and may be affected by compromised general health. There is an increased risk of HIV infection and Hepatitis B carrier status in IV drug users (Chapter 15). Gloves should be worn at all times when carrying out oral hygiene because of the risk of infection from people whose carrier status is unknown.

17.13 Personality disorders

There are no specific oral problems associated with personality disorders, although some behavioural characteristics may create barriers to seeking dental care. Sensitive and skilled handling by the dental team is necessary to establish a good relationship. Irregular dental attendance and frequent changes of dentists are the likely consequences of a poor relationship between patient and dental team. The oral side-effects of medication must be considered in relation to oral health.

17.14 People with learning difficulties

Psychiatric and behavioural disorders affect this group as they do the general population. A high rate of psychiatric disorder is reported in people with learning difficulties, particularly in those with severe impairments[31]. Oral and dental aspects are covered in Chapter 11 under developmental disorders.

17.15 Children and adolescents

The aetiology of psychiatric disease in children and adolescents is complex and multi-factorial. Behavioural problems and stress related psychiatric disorders do not of themselves produce any oral problems. Chronic or life-threatening illness may have an oral component, while behavioural problems may interfere with dental care. Attention Deficit Hyperactivity Disorder (ADHD) is common affecting 3-5% of the population, with boys affected more commonly than girls[32]. Methylphenidate hydrochloride (Ritalin, Equasym and Concerta) is frequently prescribed for the management of ADHD; one of the many side-effects is dry mouth. Other psychotropic drugs may also be prescribed. Therefore attention to oral hygiene to reduce oral side-effects is essential. Behaviour that maintains oral health is most effective when established at an early age. The reader should refer to Chapter 3 for the principles of oral care and preventive advice for children.

17.16 Summary

The objective of this chapter is to highlight the oral and dental problems associated with mental health problems. It is clear that life-style, poor motivation, impaired mental function and disturbed or psychotic behaviour have an impact on oral health. The situation is complicated by long term anti-psychotic medication which reduces salivation.

As the search continues for drugs with fewer side-effects, hopefully it will be possible to eliminate drugs with anticholinergic properties that reduce salivary secretions. With greater understanding of the causes of mental illness, and an increasing trend towards alternative therapies, the prescription of medication may decrease. The role of health care professionals is paramount in ensuring that oral and dental problems are identified, that appropriate advice and oral care are provided, and support is given to make contact with an appropriate dental service.

References

1. World Health Organisation International Classification of Mental and Behavioural Disorders. International Classification of Diseases. 10th ed. 1993.
2. Thompson D. Mental Illness: the fundamental facts. The Mental Health Foundation, 1993.
3. Mental Health Foundation Factsheets. www.mentalhealth.org.uk accessed 2004.
4. National Service Framework for Mental Health. 1999.
5. Office of Population Censuses and Surveys. People who are homeless. Mental Health Services, a place in mind. London: OPCS, 1995.
6. Angellilo IF, Nobile CGA, Pavia M et al. Dental health and treatment needs in institutionalised psychiatric patients in Italy. Community Dent Oral Epidemiol 1995 23: 360-364.

7. Hede B. Oral health in Danish hospitalised psychiatric patients. *Community Dent Oral Epidemiol* 1995 **23**: 44-48.

8. Whyman RA, Treasure ET, Brown RH *et al.* The oral health of long-term residents of a hospital for the intellectually handicapped and psychiatrically ill. *New Zealand Dent J* 1995 **91**: 49-56.

9. Blackmore T, Williams SA, Prendergast MJ *et al.* The dental health of single male hostel dwellers in Leeds. *Community Dent Health* 1995 **12**: 104-109.

10. Dicks, J. Outpatient dental services for individuals with mental illness: program description. *Spec Care Dent* 1995 **15**: 239-242.

11. Hede, B. Self -assessment of dental health among Danish non-institutionalized psychiatric patients. *Spec Care Dent* 1992 **12**: 33-36.

12. Angellilo IF, Grasso, GM, Sagliocco, G *et al.* Dental health in a group of drug addicts in Italy. *Community Dent Oral Epidemiol* 1991 **19**: 36-37.

13. Stiefel DJ, Truelove EL, Menard TW *et al.* A comparison of persons with and without chronic mental illness in community settings. *Spec Care Dent* 1990 **10**: 6-12.

14. Whittle JG, Sarll DW, Grant AA *et al.* The dental health of the elderly mentally ill: a preliminary report. *Br Dent J* 1987 **162**: 381-383.

15. British Society for Disability and Oral Health. Oral Health Care for People with Mental Health Problems: Guidelines and Recommendations. Report of BSDH Working Group. 2000. www.bsdh.org.uk

16. Nuttall NM, Bradnock G, White D *et al.* Dental attendance in 1998 and implications for the future. *Br Dent J* 2001 **190**: 177-182.

17. Locker D. Psychosocial consequences of dental fear and anxiety. *Community Dent Oral Epidemiol* 2003 **31**: 144-151.

18. Morris S, Benjamin S, Gray S *et al.* Physical, psychiatric and social characteristics of the temperomandibular disorder pain functional syndrome: the relationship of mental disorders to presentation. *Br Dent J* 1997 **182**: 255-260.

19. Scully C, Cawson RA. Psychiatric disorders. In: *Medical Problems in Dentistry.* P374-395. Oxford: Butterworth-Heineman, 1998.

20. Friedlander AH, Birch NJ. Dental conditions in patients with bipolar disorder on long-term lithium. *Spec Care Dent* 1990 **10**: 148-149.

21. Alzheimer's Disease Society. Factsheets. www.alzheimers.org.uk accessed 2004.

22. National Institute of Neurological Disorders and Strokes. Dementia with Lewy Bodies information page. 2002. www.nids.nih.gov/health

23. Chalmers JM, Carter KD, Spencer AJ. Oral diseases and conditions in community-living older adults with and without dementia. *Spec Care Dent* 2003 23: 7-17.

24. Chalmers JM, Carter KD, Spencer AJ. Caries incidence and increments in community-living older adults with and without dementia. *Gerodontology* 2002 **19**: 80-94.

25. Warren JJ, Chalmers JM, Levy SM *et al.* Oral health of persons with and without dementia attending a geriatric clinic. *Spec Care Dent* 1997 **17**: 47-53.

26. Whittle JG, Sarll DW, Grant AA *et al.* The dental health of the elderly mentally ill: the carers' perspective. *Br Dent J* 1988 **164**: 144-147.

27. Disability Discrimination Act, 1995.

28. Hugo PJ, Lacey JH. Eating disorders – diagnosis and management. *Primary Care Psych* 1996 **2**: 87-100.

29. Milosevic A. Eating disorders and the dentist. *Br Dent J* 1999 **186**: 109-113.

30. Darling MR, Arendorf TM. Review of the effects of cannabis smoking on oral health. *Int Dent J* 1992 **42**: 19-22.

31. Cooper S. Epidemiology of psychiatric disorders in elderly people compared with younger adults with learning disabilities. *Br J Psychiatry* 1997 **170**: 375-380.

32. Efron D, Kilpatrick NM. Attention Deficit Hyperactivity Disorder: A review and guide for dental professionals. *J Disabil Oral Health* 2002 **3**: 7-12.

Chapter 18

Dependence, dysphagia, critical and palliative care

18.1 Introduction

In providing or supervising oral care for dependent, unconscious, dysphagic or critically ill patients, it is essential to ensure that the airway is protected. Oral care for individuals with dysphagia (impaired swallow) requires careful management. An understanding of the mechanism of swallowing is necessary before the most appropriate and safe method of oral care can be selected. Dysphagia has many causes. It is not confined to neurological impairment but is affected by a range of other factors. Combined with cognitive impairment, dysphagia may limit the standard of oral care that can be provided. Nevertheless, oral care regimes can be adapted to accommodate individual problems and make a significant contribution to the individual's oral comfort and sense of well-being during periods of dependence and in the terminal stages of life.

18.2 Normal swallow

The process of swallowing can be divided into three phases: oral, pharyngeal and oesophageal. The oral phase is mainly voluntary; it can be initiated or arrested at will. The involuntary phase, once initiated, triggers the pharyngeal phase. Both pharyngeal and oesophageal phases are involuntary. Mastication involves complex sensory and motor function. Salivary secretion stimulated by the presence of food acts as a lubricant to facilitate mastication and swallow. When mastication is complete, the tongue, aided by oral musculature, rolls food into a bolus and pushes it towards the pharynx. Liquids are swallowed immediately and succulent foods very quickly.

Swallowing may be a function of how rapidly foods stimulate salivary flow. During this phase, lips are closed and the soft palate is lowered to protect the airway. When the tongue propels food into the pharynx, the swallow reflex, which takes approximately one second, is triggered. Once swallowing is initiated, involuntary pharyngeal and oesophageal stages continue. Breathing is temporarily arrested during the pharyngeal stage and the airway protected until the bolus reaches the oesophagus.

18.3 Dysphagia (impaired swallow)

Dysphagia may occur due to failure of one or all of the stages described and has a number of possible causes; organic causes are summarised in *Table 18.1*. Dyspahgia may occur as a complication of radical surgery for treatment of carcinoma or due to fibrosis following radiotherapy (Chapter

16). Globus hystericus is a psychogenic cause of dysphagia.

Table 18.1 Causes of dysphagia[1]

Local causes	Neurological / neuromuscular causes
Benign swellings	Achalasia
Carcinoma	Cerebellar disease
External pressure	Cerebrovascular accident
Foreign bodies	Cerebrovascular disease
Inflammatory lesions of the throat	Dermatomyositis
Paterson-Kelly syndrome	Diphtheria
Pharyngeal pouches	Guillain-Barré syndrome
Scleroderma	Motor neurone disease
Xerostomia	Multiple sclerosis
	Muscular dystrophies
	Myopathies: Myasthenia gravis
	Poliomyelitis
	Syringobulbia

The primary concern is the maintenance of nutrition and protection of the airway. If oral nutrition is inadequate, non-oral feeding is implemented alone or as a supplement to oral feeding. The risk of aspiration increases if there is:

• Impairment or delay in the involuntary phase of swallowing
• Impairment of the laryngeal protective mechanism
• Loss of sensation in the area
• Absence of cough reflex.

Problems confined to the oral voluntary stage may affect the type and quantity of nutrition. Liquids are more difficult to manage; moist pureed meals facilitate swallowing. Problems with the pharyngeal stage can cause choking, coughing and aspiration; non-oral feeding is usually implemented. Food additives e.g. modified maize starch (Thick and Easy) are used to thicken liquids to facilitate safe swallow. Most other food supplements are provided in a consistency that promotes safe swallow; as nutritional food supplements, they have a high calorific value and increase the risk of dental caries. Surgical intervention may be necessary for problems with the oesophageal stage if reflux occurs.

Factors which affect normal swallow are summarised in *Table 18.2*. The infantile swallow is characterised by a tongue thrust. Primitive oral reflexes may develop as a result of cortical deficit and cranial nerve involvement;

tongue thrust and bite reflex pose problems for oral care. A swallow assessment is essential to identify the type and degree of dysphagia and the intactness of the cough reflex before planning oral care techniques. Interdisciplinary assessment involving speech and language therapy (SALT), physiotherapy and dietetics provides the necessary information for the management of oral care. Desensitisation techniques to promote oro-muscular activity may be recommended by SALT.

Table 18.2 Factors that affect swallowing

· Ability to form lip seal	· Underactive and hyperactive gag reflex
· Loss of sensation	· Delayed oral swallow
· Primitive oral reflexes	· Reduced awareness of food residues

Drooling (sialorrhea) is generally caused by the inability to retain saliva in the oral cavity and to coordinate the swallow mechanism rather than of excessive salivation. It may be due to any of the factors in *Table 18.2*, as well as to tongue thrust, neuromuscular in-coordination, structural abnormalities, intra-oral irritation or posture. Profuse drooling can cause peri-oral maceration, skin chapping and infection. It can also lead to social embarrassment and exclusion, and if profuse, it requires frequent changes of clothing. Factors that exacerbate drooling (sialorrhea) are listed in *Table 18.3*.

Table 18.3 Factors that may exacerbate drooling (sialorrhea)

· Head and neck position and control	· Sitting posture
· Ability to concentrate	· Emotional state
· Tongue size and position	· General health
· Obstructed nasal airway	· Oral habits
· Persistent mouth breathing	· Medication
· Dental disease (caries, periodontal status)	· Malocclusion
· Decreased oral sensory awareness[2,3].	

Approaches to improving saliva control include the elimination of aggravating factors, behavioural techniques, eating and drinking skills, oro-facial exercises and appliances, and pharmacological or surgical treatments[3]. Anticholinergic control of drooling needs to be monitored so that it does not cause dry mouth. Surgical redirection of the salivary ducts, removal of salivary glands and other more complex techniques are described but appear to have limitations[4].

Palatal training and other appliances are used with varying degrees of success in the management of dysphagia, speech disorders and drooling; improvements in swallow are reported in rehabilitation following stroke, in drooling in neurologically impaired children, and in muscular dystrophy[5-8]. A range of appliances and techniques exist for dealing with these complex problems[2].

The use of feeding plates and other pre-surgical appliances to manage feeding difficulties in babies with cleft lip and palate is controversial[9], however there is no method of assessing whether the problem being treated would have resolved without therapy.

Swallowing is difficult if the mandible cannot be stabilised. Therefore improving the retention and stability of dentures can make an important contribution to safe swallowing. Temporary or permanent relines and denture fixative are commonly used to improve denture stability. Prostheses may be designed, or dentures modified to support musculature by eliminating the sulcus on the paralysed side. This increases denture stability and food is prevented from accumulating on the affected side[5]. However, loss of neuromuscular control and sensation of the oral and facial muscles can have a negative prognosis for success in wearing dentures. It is important that the dentist, patient and carer review the benefits of continued use versus the abandonment of dentures[5].

Oral health may be at risk because of a number of factors (*Table 18.4*). Calculus (*Figure 1.5*) forms significantly faster in tube-fed individuals, and therefore plaque removal is a priority[10]. Individual oro-dental assessment may offer alternative management strategies, as well as identifying oral hygiene needs in dysphagia.

Table 18.4 Factors that influence oral health

* Lack of oro-muscular control	*	Poor lip posture
* Increased tooth / food contact time	*	Mouth-breathing
* Dietary changes	*	Xerostomia
* Food accumulation due to sensory or motor loss		

18.4 Oral care for dependent or dysphagic patients

Posture is important in facilitating swallow and protecting the airway during oral care; if possible, the subject should be seated upright with feet firmly on the ground. Tilting the head backwards hinders safe swallow; a slight increase in flexion is recommended. If the subject is confined to bed, the head should be tilted forward; if reclining, the subject's head should be tilted to one side to assist drainage. With unilateral facial paralysis, the head should be tilted away from the affected side.

Whenever possible, oral care should be provided from behind the subject (*Figure 18.1*). In people with cerebral palsy, loss of neck support and movement of the head from the midline will trigger the tonic labyrinthine and asymmetrical tonic neck reflexes respectively. These reflexes can be minimised by supporting and cradling the head and neck from behind the subject. In some people with CP, it may be easier to provide oral care in the prone position.

Oral assessment (Chapter 6) identifies the type of oral care that is appropriate to the individual, should be completed by nurses on admission and evaluated regularly to review changes in oral health status and oral hygiene needs. Nurses are recommended to routinely inspect the mouth with a pen torch and spatula prior to providing oral care. Subjective assessment of oral comfort should be included. Recommendations for assessment and practical oral care are summarised in Chapter 6 and in BSDH guidelines[11]. Oral care for the dependent patient is summarised in *Tables 18.5* and *18.6*. Techniques to support physical intervention when more than one person is required to provide oral hygiene have been risk assessed[12]. Guidance on the legal and ethical issues for intervening in oral hygiene are addressed in a BSDH policy document[13].

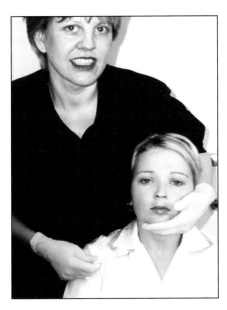

Figure 18.1
Whenever possible, oral care should be provided from behind the subject

Table 18.5 Summary of oral care for the dependent patient[11]

Prepare appropriate oral hygiene materials

Place patient in a sitting or semi-fowler's position to protect airway

Protect clothing

Remove dentures or other removable appliances

* **Dentate patient**

    If necessary, insert a prop to gain access to the mouth

    Floss interproximal surfaces of teeth, taking care not to traumatise gingivae or use an interdental brush

    Brush all surfaces using Fluoride toothpaste or chlorhexidine gel

    Rinse or aspirate to remove saliva and toothpaste residue

Remember that traditional foaming agents in toothpaste inactivate chlorhexidine so use one or other, or alternate their use at different times of the day.

* **Dentate and edentulous patients**

    Gently retract cheeks and brush inside surfaces with soft gentle strokes

    Using gauze to hold the tongue, gently pull the tongue forward and brush surface gently from rear to front

    Gently brush palate

    Towel or swab if tooth-brushing is not possible

    Aspirate throughout procedures if airway is at risk

* **Dentures and removable appliances**

    Brush vigorously with unperfumed household soap

    Pay particular attention to clasps

    Rinse well in cold water

    Saliva substitute may be required before replacing denture in the mouth

* **Intubated patients**

    Reposition tube frequently

    Ensure tube is secure before proceeding with oral care

    Proceed with oral care as appropriate.

Reproduced with kind permission of Professor June Nunn, Editor of the *Journal of Disability and Oral Health*

Table 18.6

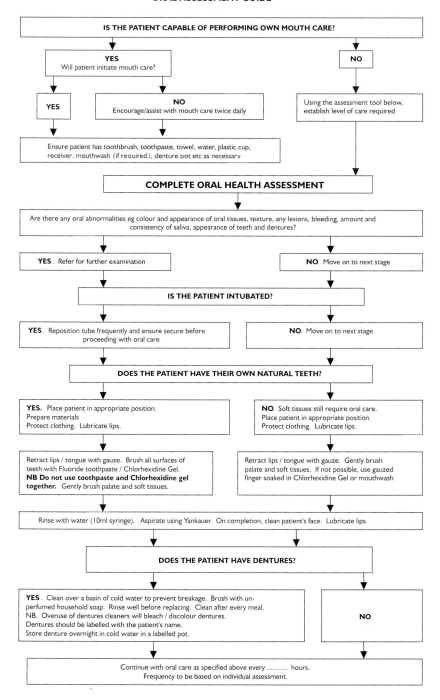

ORAL ASSESSMENT GUIDE [11]

IS THE PATIENT CAPABLE OF PERFORMING OWN MOUTH CARE?

YES
Will patient initiate mouth care?

NO

YES

NO
Encourage/assist with mouth care twice daily

Using the assessment tool below, establish level of care required

Ensure patient has toothbrush, toothpaste, towel, water, plastic cup, receiver, mouthwash (if required), denture pot etc as necessary

COMPLETE ORAL HEALTH ASSESSMENT

Are there any oral abnormalities eg colour and appearance of oral tissues, texture, any lesions, bleeding, amount and consistency of saliva, appearance of teeth and dentures?

YES. Refer for further examination

NO. Move on to next stage

IS THE PATIENT INTUBATED?

YES. Reposition tube frequently and ensure secure before proceeding with oral care

NO. Move on to next stage

DOES THE PATIENT HAVE THEIR OWN NATURAL TEETH?

YES. Place patient in appropriate position. Prepare materials Protect clothing. Lubricate lips.

NO. Soft tissues still require oral care. Place patient in appropriate position. Protect clothing. Lubricate lips.

Retract lips / tongue with gauze. Brush all surfaces of teeth with Fluoride toothpaste / Chlorhexidine Gel. **NB Do not use toothpaste and Chlorhexidine gel together.** Gently brush palate and soft tissues.

Retract lips / tongue with gauze. Gently brush palate and soft tissues. If not possible, use gauzed finger soaked in Chlorhexidine Gel or mouthwash

Rinse with water (10ml syringe). Aspirate using Yankauer. On completion, clean patient's face. Lubricate lips.

DOES THE PATIENT HAVE DENTURES?

YES. Clean over a basin of cold water to prevent breakage. Brush with un-perfumed household soap. Rinse well before replacing. Clean after every meal. NB. Overuse of dentures cleaners will bleach / discolour dentures. Dentures should be labelled with the patient's name. Store denture overnight in cold water in a labelled pot.

NO

Continue with oral care as specified above every .... hours. Frequency to be based on individual assessment.

Reproduced with kind permission of Professor June Nunn, Editor of the *Journal of Disability and Oral Health*

18.5 Oral hygiene equipment and materials

These are summarised in Chapter 9. In severe dysphagia, high volume aspiration is essential to protect the airway and ensure that toothpaste is not retained in the mouth; an aspirating toothbrush may be beneficial (*Figure 9.6*).

In contrast to most toothpastes, chlorhexidine gel does not foam, and provides the benefits of chemical plaque control. Gauze swabs soaked in chlorhexidine gel or mouthwash provide an alternative when toothbrushing cannot be achieved. Foam swabs are no substitute for a toothbrush[14]. If foam swabs were as effective as toothbrushes, they would be marketed widely for oral hygiene. Foam swabs may have some benefit in lubricating a patient's mouth but they are hazardous if the foam head becomes detached. The cost of providing a toothbrush, which can last up to 3 months, compares very favourably with the cost of a fresh daily supply of foam swabs or mouth packs (*Figure 18.2*).

For post-surgical oral care, the type and frequency of post-operative oral care is under the direction of the oral surgery or maxillo-facial team. In post-surgical and maxillary fixation, chlorhexidine is essential to maintain plaque control. Straws can be used to deliver mouthwash provided that the patient is not dysphagic. Oral irrigation devices with aspiration are beneficial and can be used to deliver lubrication and mouthwashes (Chapter 9). The mouth and fixed appliances should be cleaned with a soft toothbrush; chlorhexidine may be preferable to toothpaste based on individual assessment. Chlorhexidine spray as an alternative method of plaque control

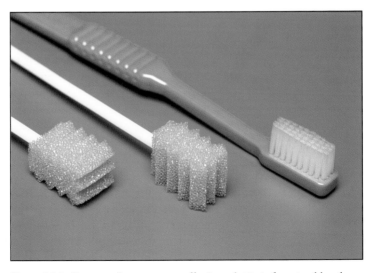

Figure 18.2 Foam swabs are not an effective substitute for a toothbrush

'reaches the parts that cannot be reached' when standard oral hygiene techniques cannot be completed, but not if the swallow is impaired.

Dentures should be removed and cleaned as directed (Chapter 2). All oral soft tissues should be brushed with a small headed soft/medium toothbrush. Only if toothbrushing cannot be achieved should towelling or swabbing be used as a substitute. Saliva substitutes may be necessary to alleviate xerostomia (Chapter 9). Dry and crusted lips may be bathed with saline and lubricated with an emollient; KY jelly is recommended[15]. Dietary adjustment should take account of the risk of caries from extrinsic sugars for dentate patients.

18.6 Palliative oral care

Palliative care is defined as 'the total active care of patients whose disease is not responsive to treatment'. Control of pain, of other symptoms, and of psychological, social and spiritual problems is paramount. The goal of palliative care is achievement of the best quality of life for patients and their families. Many aspects of palliative care are also applicable earlier in the course of illness in conjunction with anti-cancer treatment (Chapter 16).

The priority is to provide comfort and relief of painful and distressing oral symptoms in prolonging active life and in the terminal stages of life. Subjective assessment is even more important and oral hygiene techniques should be modified according to reported symptom relief. Regular re-assessment of oral status and evaluation of techniques and materials used for oral care are central to effective palliative oral care.

Oral health in palliative care is receiving greater attention. Common oral symptoms include pain, soreness, ulceration, glossitis, candidal infections, and dry mouth (xerostomia), symptoms that have a serious impact on quality of life. A study of hospice patients confirms the high number with oral symptoms[16], in which 50% had some degree of gingival inflammation and other oral pathologies. Of the 75% wearing dentures, 71% had denture problems and 60% wore their dentures at night. Many dentures were old and unsatisfactory due to the wearer's weight loss, and yet denture relines provided at the bedside can offer rapid relief and a solution to poor fit. Oral complications are reported among significant numbers of terminally ill cancer patients; 97% complained of oral dryness and on examination, 90% had clinically dry mouths (xerostomia)[17]. Oral fungal infections, mainly candida are common[18], while herpes simplex is frequently re-activated in patients with advanced carcinoma. Furthermore, pain relief with opiate derivatives exacerbates xerostomia and other oral pathology.

Oral care regimes are based on the relief and improvement of symptoms. The principles are summarised in *Table 18.7*. Many of the symptoms can be alleviated by maintaining oral cleanliness, adequate lubrication and anti-fungal antibiotic therapy. Mouthwashes and swabbing may be more appropriate than a toothbrush to care for friable oral tissues. The taste of chlorhexidine 0.2% (Corsodyl) may be unacceptable as it can induce a burning sensation. Chlorhexidine 0.1% mouthwash (Eludril) is less effective but may be better tolerated. Povidone-Idodine (Betadine) is an alternative but mucosal irritation and hypersensitivity reactions are reported. Benzydamine hydrochloride (Difflam), an anti-inflammatory containing topical analgesia can provide pain relief for sore mouth; used prior to eating, it is effective in alleviating mild to moderate mucositis. Treatment of fungal infections can present management problems due to drug resistance and potential drug interactions; systemic anti-fungals may be required. Herpes simplex should be treated with systemic acyclovir pending confirmation by culture. Maintaining lubrication and alleviating dry mouth are essential. Detailed regimes that rely on oral and subjective assessment, techniques and materials are also covered in other chapters.

In childhood, the principles of palliative care are based on adequately controlling symptoms of pain, anorexia, nausea and vomiting, constipation, weakness and lassitude. Oral problems are treated routinely with chlorhexidine, appropriate anti-fungals, lignocaine ointment, benzydamine hydrochloride and tender loving care. The involvement of suitably trained dental professionals is essential in order to ensure that oral care protocols are appropriate[19].

The effects on the oral cavity of malignant disease and its treatment are discussed in Chapter 16. Deaths in hospice care are mainly due to malignancy, and oral symptoms are both common and distressing. The importance of oral health care is often overlooked due to the omission of the dentist as a member of the palliative care team. The case for including a dentist in the palliative care team is undeniable in order to ensure that oro-dental needs are managed effectively[20].

Table 18.7 Principles of palliative care

* Removal of plaque and food debris
* Denture hygiene and use
* Relief of xerostomia
* Relief of other reported symptoms

18.7   Summary

This chapter summarises the principles of oral care for people who are largely dependent on others for oral care and who require professional support for the relief of distressing oral symptoms. The contents are of particular importance for the professional nurse. Although there are clear medical imperatives for effective oral care to minimise the effects of oral and dental disease, an additional objective is the reduction of discomfort and improved quality of life for people undergoing painful and distressing treatment regimes. To be able to eat and drink comfortably are basic human needs that are even more important for people with a debilitating or terminal condition.

If there is one connecting theme running through Section 3, it is the need for close collaboration between all members of the health care team and the dental team. Although it is the primary health care professional who will be helping the patient with day-to-day maintenance of oral health, it is the authors' contention that this task can be supported and augmented by working closely with the dental team.

References

1. Scully C, Cawson RA. Gastrointestinal disorders. In: *Medical Problems in Dentistry.* P184-185. Oxford: Butterworth-Heineman, 1998.

2. Andersson-Norinder J, Sjogreen L. Orofacial dysfunction *In Disability and Oral Care.* pp 104-114. Ed J Nunn. London: FDI World Dental Press Ltd., 2000.

3. Kilpatrick NM, Johnson H, Reddihough D. Sialorrhea: a multidisciplinary approach to the management of drooling children. *J Disabil Oral Health* 2000 **1:** 3-9.

4. Tahmassebi JF, Curzon MEJ. Evaluation of the outcome of different management approaches to reduce drooling in children with cerebral palsy. *J Disabil Oral Health* 2003 **4:** 19-25.

5. White SM. Denture treatment for the stroke patient. *Br Med J* 1997 **183:** 179-184.

6. Selley WG, Roche MT, Pearce VR *et al.* Dysphagia following strokes: clinical observations of swallowing rehabilitation employing palatal training appliances. *Dysphagia* 1995 **10:** 32-35.

7. Lloyd-Faulconbridge RV, Tranter RM, Moffat V *et al.* Review of management of drooling problems in neurologically impaired children: a review of methods and results over 6 years at Chailey Heritage Clinical Services. *Clin Otolaryngol* 2001 **26:** 76-81.

8. Day CJ, Welbury RR. Treatment of drooling in congenital muscular dystrophy with a palatal training appliance. *J Disabil Oral Health* 2000 **1:** 10-12.

9. Rivkin CJ, Keith O, Crawford PJM *et al.* Dental care for the patient with a cleft lip and palate. Part I: From birth to the mixed dentition stage. *Br Dent J* 2000 **188:** 78-83.

10. Dicks JL, Banning JS. Evaluation of calculus accumulation in tube-fed mentally handicapped patients: the effects of oral hygiene status. *Spec Care Dent* 1991 **11:** 104-106.

11. Griffiths J, Lewis D. Guidelines for the oral care of patients who are dependent, dysphagic or critically ill. *J Disabil Oral Health* 2002 **3:** 30-33.

12. Griffiths JE, Campiutti T, Habbijam E *et al.* A pilot study to address barriers to physical intervention for oral hygiene. Abstracts 16th Congress of the International Association for Disability and Oral Health. 2002; 42.

13. British Society for Disability and Oral Health. Principles on intervention for people unable to comply with routine dental care. A Policy document. 2004. www.bsdh.org.uk

14. Bowsher J, Boyle S, Griffiths J. A clinical effectiveness systematic review of oral care. *Nursing Standard* 1999 **13:** 31.

15. British Society for Disability and Oral Health. Guidelines for the oral management of oncology patients requiring radiotherapy, chemotherapy and bone marrow transplantation. *J Disabil Oral Health* 2001 **2:** 3-14.

16. Aldred MJ, Addy M, Bagg J *et al.* Oral health in the terminally ill: a cross-sectional pilot survey. *Spec Care Dent* 1991 **11:** 59-62.

17. Sweeney MP, Bagg J, Baxter WP *et al.* Oral disease in terminally ill cancer patients with xerostomia. *Oral Oncol* 1998 **34:** 123-126.

18. Bagg J, Sweeney MP, Lewis MA *et al.* High prevalence of non-albicans yeasts and detection of anti-fungal resistance in the oral flora of patients with advanced cancer. *Palliat Med* 2003 **17:** 477-482.

19. Collard MM, Hunter ML. Oral care protocols for children receiving treatment for cancer. *J Disabil Oral Health* 2001 **2:** 15-17.

20. Wiseman MA. Palliative Care Dentistry. *Gerodontology* 2000 **17:** 49-51.

Section 4: Oral health promotion

This section looks at some of the current approaches to health promotion and some practical applications for oral health promotion. It is aimed at the primary healthcare worker whose role includes promoting, improving and maintaining their clients' oral health. The contents of this section will also be useful for workers involved in teaching and training oral health educators.

All health workers, potentially, have a role in promoting health but this often has a lower priority in comparison to treatment and care. This is also the case for oral health. Pressures on time, resources and the way the health services are organised can make it difficult to devote adequate time to promoting health and prevention. A focus on short-term results in the planning of health services also does not encourage health promotion, where changes in practices can take many years. Many health workers used to receive minimal or no training in effective health promotion skills during their primary training, which left them ill-equipped.

However there have been recent changes in global and government policies that are placing the promotion of health in a more important position[1]. This has lead to programmes to tackle the causes of ill health and inequalities. Many health workers now have an increased emphasis on health promotion in their training and it forms part of their continuing education.

Even though there are overall improvements in the oral health of the population[2], oral and dental diseases continue to cause much suffering. This results in a significant drain on the resources of health care systems. The effects of oral disease can range from significant embarrassment in social interactions to impairing conditions that affect the quality of life[3].

Methods of preventing oral disease are quite simple and have been reiterated throughout this book:

- Restrict sugar intake as part of a healthy diet
- Practice effective oral hygiene
- Use fluoride products
- Avoid smoking
- Maintain regular dental attendance.

There are still difficulties for significant sections of society to practice these approaches and the role of the oral health promoter is to support people to maintain their own oral health. It is our view that one of the reasons is that oral and dental health have been outside the mainstream of health promotion and kept as a speciality for dental teams. The lack of training in oral and dental disease in the curricula of most primary health care professionals is an issue we hope this book will address and Chapter 20 describes some of the practical approaches that can be used to deliver effective oral health education and health promotion programmes.

It is now well recognised that a 'common risk' approach to tackling oral disease is more effective[4]. We are advocating that oral health promotion is an integral part of primary health care and not just the domain of the dental team. The core knowledge of oral health required by a health promoter is contained in Section 1 of this text and is based around The Scientific Basis of Oral Health Education[5]. As people receive their oral health knowledge from a variety of sources, often commercial or anecdotal, a grounding in the core, evidence based knowledge areas is very important to help individuals make the right decisions.

There are no real differences in the skills needed for oral health promotion. These include:

- Teaching
- Counselling
- Demonstrating
- Empowering
- Lobbying
- Networking.

Extensive skills in oral diagnosis and treatment are not required provided access to professional dental services are available. In most industrialised countries this is less of a problem than in developing countries where the primary health care professional may also have to provide more clinical oral services.

References

1. Ewles L, Simnett I. Promoting Health. A Practical Guide. 4th Ed. pxxi. Baillière Tindall. 1999.
2. Nuttall N, Steele JG, Nunn J et al. A Guide to the UK Adult Dental Health Survey 1998. p1. London: BDA Books, 2001.
3. Nuttall N, Steele JG, Nunn J et al. A Guide to the UK Adult Dental Health Survey 1998. p29. London: BDA Books, 2001.
4. Sheiham A, Watt RG. The common risk approach: a rational basis for promoting oral health. *Community Dent Oral Epidemiol* 2000 28:399-406.

5. Levine R, Stillman-Lowe C. The scientific basis of oral health education. 5th Edition. London: British Dental Association, 2004.

Chapter 19

Approaches to health promotion

19.1   Introduction

This chapter examines aspects of health and health status and how oral health is integrated into these approaches. The way in which illness affects behaviour and the ability to function is examined to give some insight into effective interventions.

19.2   What is health and oral health?

Health for many people is a useful social product, a tool to help them with day-to-day living. It is often taken for granted until symptoms or an illness prevents them from doing something. It can be viewed as having a positive or negative meaning. The positive definition, as a state of well being is encapsulated in the WHO definition as:

" A state of complete physical, mental and social well being, not merely the absence of disease or infirmity" (WHO 1946)[1].

This definition is now viewed as being idealistic as it is difficult to imagine how anyone can reach 'a complete state'. It does not recognise that people will define their own views of health and that conditions change.

A negative definition of health is the absence of disease or illness. This approach is used predominantly in the training of many health professionals. As the health profession has considerable status in society, this approach is influential. It has been challenged as being too focussed on the treatment of disease rather than the prevention and ignoring the effects of social factors such as housing, sanitation, education and wealth.

A more holistic concept of health describes six dimensions of health[2]:

- Physical health
- Mental health
- Emotional health
- Social health
- Spiritual health
- Societal health.

The first five components are individually based, the sixth recognising that it is difficult to be healthy in a 'sick' society. The dimensions are inter-linked and often the boundaries blur in day-to-day life. It is the contention of the authors that there is little value in considering oral health as different to general health. Good oral health is something that is expressed often in purely functional terms:

- Freedom from pain and discomfort
- An ability to eat and speak
- Acceptable appearance.

Oral and dental diseases are very widespread but it is only when they impinge on any of the three above criteria that they become issues.

19.3   Health promotion and primary health care

The main approaches to health care in the last few decades have been shaped by the Primary Health Care Approach (PHCA)[3]. This has refocussed the approach to illness and disease from purely treatment to include preventive and rehabilitation aspects based on health promotion. The PHCA has been driven by policies at a global level from the WHO and basically entails that health workers are not just in the business of providing health care for people, they are also involved with helping people to do it themselves.

The Ottawa Charter for health promotion states:

"Health promotion is the process of enabling people to increase control over, and to improve, their health. To reach a stage of complete physical, mental and social well being an individual or group must be able to identify and realise aspirations, to satisfy needs and to change or cope with the environment".[4]

How and where health workers get involved in health promotion will vary. Certainly, health promotion is not purely the domain of health care organisations, it involves governments at a local and national level, local authorities and the voluntary sector. The primary health care team has an expanding role, particularly with health education, prevention and maximising peoples' potential for self care. Chapter 20 describes in more detail some of the activities not only with individuals and families but also with the teaching and training of other agencies.

19.4   Helping people to make healthy choices

Many of the causes of ill health have been attributed to peoples' behaviour and their lifestyles. Health promotion approaches often involve working on changes and helping people make healthier choices. The choices that people make are also strongly affected by the environment in which they live and often their living conditions and socio-economic conditions affect their ability to make changes but there is often potential for some change. To maximise healthy changes it is important for the health promoter to have an understanding why people behave in particular ways and some of the processes involved in how people change. An effective health promoter needs a range of skills and knowledge to support people change. These include:

- Knowledge of how to effectively prevent disease and ill health
- Skills in teaching and education to transfer that knowledge
- Understanding of health behaviour and how people change.

In recent years, the basics of social psychology have been included in the training of many health workers to equip them with the basic toolkit to be effective health promoters. Changing health behaviour is not easy or based on a quick decision either for the individual or for the health promoter.

19.5   Health behaviour

This section examines some of the basics of health behaviour from the perspective of social psychology. A person's behaviour is partly influenced by their attitude towards that behaviour. An attitude is influenced by beliefs, and the motivation to act, which in turn comes from a person's values, drives and the influences from social norms. These components of health behaviour are often formed in early life and influenced by the family and later by other significant people in an individual's life.

Beliefs
A belief is based on the knowledge a person has about something. This can be positive. For example, exercise is good; or negative, for example, sugar is bad for teeth. A person's beliefs can be strongly influenced by information but that alone does not always result in a change in behaviour. For example, the risks of smoking are well known but a sizeable portion of the population start and continue to smoke.

Values
Values are more emotionally laden beliefs and are derived from mixing with family, friends and peers. They describe those things that a person thinks are important, for example, good dental health is important.

Attitudes
Attitudes are more specific than values and do not tend to change easily.

An attitude is made up of a person's knowledge and their feelings of what is important. As they are so resistant to change, an attitude can change behaviour and once changed may influence attitude change. An often cited example is the strong anti-smoking attitudes sometimes adopted by ex-smokers.

Drives

A drive is a strong motivating factor. This may be hunger, thirst, sex, pain, addiction and other basic needs. Sometimes these are even at the level of basic instincts and can override beliefs and attitudes. It is difficult to make healthy choices if these basic drives have not been met. The next stage in the toolkit of social psychology is a study of how all these factors come together in the form of models. There are a number of examples in current use. One of the most useful is a model of how people change.

The Stages of Change Model

As we have seen, changing behaviour is a complex process. This model, from the work of Prochaska and DiClemente[5] describes various stages of change. It shows that change is a cycle, not a one-way process, *Figure 19.1* depicts the model. The various stages of change include:

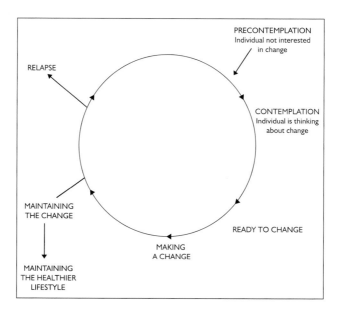

Figure 19.1 The stages of change model (after Prochaska and DiClemente). Reproduced from Naidoo and Wills. Health Promotion. Foundations for Practice. 2nd Ed p31 1999 with kind permission of Elsevier[5]

Pre-contemplation

At this early stage a person has not considered changing their lifestyle or even that there are risks in their health behaviour.

Contemplation

An individual may be aware of the benefits of change but are not yet ready for change. Often information or help may be needed to make the decision to progress to the next stage.

Preparing to change

As the benefits of change are now seen to outweigh the costs and the conditions are ready, the individual may be ready to change with support.

Change

In the early stage of change the individual needs to make a definite decision to do things differently. They will need clear goals, support and rewards.

Maintenance

The new behaviour is now maintained and the person is living a healthier lifestyle. At this stage it is possible to relapse and move back to earlier stages. But because the process is seen as a cycle, this is not seen as a complete failure. An individual will move backwards and forwards through the cycle.

An example often used is smoking. As part of the process of change to a non-smoker a person may have several relapses at the 'change-maintenance' phase. At different stages the interventions needed will also be different. In the earlier stages a person may require information in order to decide to change. At a later stage, support with formulating a plan. At the actual stage of change, support may include interventions and counselling. The help for people who have relapsed will be quite different to support at the move to change for the first time. The value of using this type of approach is in the following key areas:

- Involving the client in the change process which has a greater chance of success
- It recognises that change is a process, not a single decision
- It helps the health promoter identify the appropriate help at key stages.

For more a more detailed look at models on health behaviour the Further

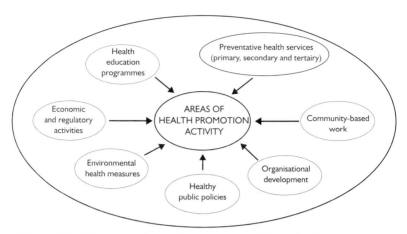

Figure 19.2 A framework for health promotion activities (after Ewles and Simnett). Reproduced from Ewles and Simnett Promoting Health. A practical Guide 4th Ed. p30 1999 with kind permission of Elsevier[8]

Reading section (Appendix 3) of this book will be useful.

19.6   Health promotion activities

A traditional approach to promoting health has been mainly concerned with education of the individual and the preventive activities of the health professional. This tends to focus on the individual and their families and ignores the wider influences on health. Ewles and Simnett have proposed a more comprehensive approach which focuses on the concept of health gain[6]. The term 'health gain' was first used in Wales in the strategic approaches to planning health services[6]. The term was later used in the rest of the UK and the WHO. A useful working definition of health gain is:[7]

"A measurable improvement in health status, in an individual or population, attributable to earlier intervention."

If the aim of our interventions are to improve health, a useful model of activities shown in *Figure 19.2* demonstrates the range of activities that are needed.[8] There are several categories of activity which involve the health worker and many other agencies working together. Health workers are not just limited to working within preventive health services and health education programmes, but will find that there are areas of overlap.

19.7   Oral health promotion activities

If we examine the different categories in the model of activities described by Ewles and Simnett[8], we can identify some actions for oral health promoters. To be most effective, most of these activities should take place in an integrated approach with other agencies.

Preventive health services
Preventive services often involve the direct activities of health professionals. Some of the more obvious examples in primary dental care include:

- Fisssure sealants
- Scaling and polishing teeth
- Fluoride applications
- Screening of groups and populations
- Denture cleaning and naming
- Provision of mouth guards.

Health education programmes
Health education can take place in a formal programme and location in:

- One-to-one situations in clinics and surgeries
- Groups in schools, clubs and centres

This group of activities involves lobbying, political and educational activity directed towards politicians, policy makers and planners on a range of issues including:

- Sugar advertising
- Water fluoridation
- Tobacco taxation
- Food labelling
- Improving access to dental services.

This is closely linked, and will frequently overlap with:

- Policies on healthy eating at national level and local level
- Improving access to oral health products
- Improving choice in vending machines
- Smoke free areas
- Training in oral care skills for health and care workers.

Community based work

There is an increasing role of the oral health promoter working with community development teams. The focus is working with people to identify and take action for themselves. Although this may not have an initial oral health focus, a wider holistic approach will benefit oral health indirectly.

19.8 Summary

- We have demonstrated that health promotion is an integral part of primary health care
- We have examined some aspects of health behaviour and how people can make changes
- We have described how oral health promotion should be integrated into health promotion activities.

References

1. World Health Organisation (1948) in Ewles L and Simnett I. *Promoting Health. A Practical Guide.* 4th Ed. p19. Baillière Tindall, 1999.

2. Ewles L, Simnett I. *Promoting Health. A Practical Guide.* 4th Ed. p7. Baillière Tindall, 1999.

3. WHO (1978). Alma Ata 1978: Primary Health Care. (Health for All Series No.1).

4. World Health Organisation (1986) in Ewles L and Simnett I. *Promoting Health. A Practical Guide.* 4th Ed. p14. Baillière Tindall, 1999.

5. Prochaska J.O, DiClemente CC (1986). Towards a comprehensive model of change. In Naidoo J and Wills J. *Health Promotion. Foundations for Practice.* 2nd Ed. p231. Baillière Tindall, 2000.

6. Ewles L, Simnett I. *Promoting Health. A Practical Guide.* 4th Ed. p24. Baillière Tindall, 1999.

7. Ibid, p25.

8. Ibid, p30.

Chapter 20

Practical oral health promotion

20.1   Introduction

This chapter looks at practical ways in which oral health promotion can be undertaken. The emphasis is on interventions that are effective, as supported by research evidence[1,2] and conform to sound health promotion principles.

20.2   Oral health promotion throughout life

An individual goes through a life career in certain roles:

- Dependant pre-school child
- School student
- Adult with differing roles including, parent and carer
- Older age.

As an individual passes through these stages, he or she is more amenable at the time of transition to change, as part of taking on the new role. However, as an individual does not exist in a vacuum but is part of a family, community and other groups, they will also be affected by health promotion approaches initially targeted at those nearby.

20.3   Approaches to oral health promotion

Although there has been a decline in dental caries, described in Chapter 1, it still presents a considerable problem for the whole community. The reduction in new dental disease is seen throughout the whole population and it is important not just to target the sectors where the levels are highest[3].

The risk factors for oral and dental disease are the same as for many chronic conditions and include:

- Diet
- Hygiene
- Smoking
- Alcohol use
- Stress
- Trauma.

It is more logical to approach oral health promotion in collaboration with other health promotion initiatives to provide a more holistic approach. A whole community approach, addressing a range of risk factors is the preferred approach.

20.4 Choosing effective approaches

There have been two major reviews of the effectiveness of approaches to oral health promotion[1,2] and both have examined the published research evidence based on clinical effectiveness. However it should be noted that the reviews are in some ways historical as they examined research already published, sometimes several decades ago. Many of the papers examined did not meet the more current very high standards for modern research and were descriptive of the interventions without demonstrating any clear outcomes. In many respects the reviews are useful in demonstrating the previous shortcomings of earlier programmes and later in this chapter the way forward is considered. As most of the oral health outcomes of health promotion interventions cannot be demonstrated in the short term or even attributed to one particular intervention, it is important to plan interventions with clear aims and objectives. A range of short- term goals can be identified to help evaluate effectiveness.

20.5 Main findings of the effectiveness reviews

Some of the key main findings of the major reviews are listed below, although it will be of value to examine the full reviews when planning oral health promotion interventions.

- Oral health promotion, which includes the use of fluoride, is effective in reducing caries
- School based health education aimed at improving oral hygiene has not been shown to be effective, dental clinic based oral hygiene measures can be effective
- Oral health promotion aimed at improving oral hygiene using simple approaches can reduce dental plaque levels
- Oral health promotion can improve knowledge levels but this is not necessarily linked to changes in behaviour
- The effects of oral health promotion on attitude change are unclear at this stage.[1]
- It is unclear whether one-off initiatives will improve oral health for long periods
- More innovative approaches can produce longer term behaviour change
- Limited short term changes can be achieved using simple approaches

- All ages are able to benefit from effective health promotion programmes although elderly people may require more support than younger people

- Longer term health gains are possible if the social environments of the very young are targeted.[2]

20.6   Planning oral health promotion

The key to effective health promotion lies in effective planning. Oral health promotion interventions are often initiated in response to a national initiative to improve health. These can arise from a government level strategy to address inequalities in health e.g. Better Health Wales[4], or Our Healthier Nation[5]. These high level strategies will set key targets and direct funding towards initiatives. However many of the targets will be comparatively short term as they fit in with the political cycle. Strategies such as these are also focussed on some of the major causes of mortality such as coronary health disease and cancers. This can mean that issues such as oral health appear lower priority. However it is our contention that well-planned oral health promotion programmes demonstrating clear

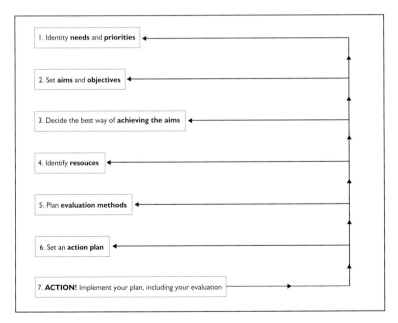

Figure 20.1
A flowchart for planning and evaluating health promotion (after Ewles and Simnett)[6]
Reproduced from Ewles and Simnett Promoting Health. A practical guide. 4th Ed p27
1999 with kind permission of Elsevier

objectives in short and long term that demonstrate how resources are used effectively can be commissioned in the competitive process of allocating funding.

Ewles and Simnett[6] describe a very useful seven-stage planning and evaluation cycle that can be used to produce effective oral health promotion interventions *Figure 20.1*. This planning process should be used for all types of interventions, small and large, short and long term. There is always an inclination to start the intervention as soon as possible in order that some early successes can be demonstrated. The short-term nature of the funding can also be a temptation for early action. Before commencing action the following three journey-related questions should be answered:

- Where am I going?
- How will I get there?
- How will I know when I am there?

The first question is concerned with the first two steps shown in *Figure 20.1*; identifying needs and priorities and setting aims and objectives. The second question is covered by steps 3 and 4; deciding the best way of achieving the aims and identifying the resources. The final question is related to the process of evaluation. In many ways the most important reason for a planning process is to ensure that effective evaluation is included. The traditional approach to evaluation was to only consider it after the intervention, more of a post-mortem approach.

The approach described by Ewles and Simnett highlights that the whole planning process is a cyclical one, including constant reviewing and changing, and most importantly, thinking about evaluation at all stages.

Using a cyclical approach to planning will also recognise that in the real world we rarely commence at step 1 but often have to respond to an idea or strategy or a call for projects related to specific funding and commence planning from that point.

20.7 Settings for oral health promotion

In the Introductory section to this chapter we described some opportunities during an individual's life when changes can be made. The settings for oral health promotion to work with individuals and those around them at those stages include:

- Oral health promotion in neighbourhoods

- Oral health promotion in schools
- Oral health promotion in the workplace
- Oral health promotion in primary health care and hospitals.

Focussing the approaches for oral health promotion on a settings approach is one that is advocated by the World Health Organisation. The Ottawa Charter[8] highlights the importance of settings as ' health is created and lived by people within the settings of their everyday life; where they learn, work, play and love.' This is a development of the traditional, medical model approach to focussing on diseases and health problems. A further advantage of a settings approach is that it will encourage a wider approach to health promotion, away from just individual-based health education. The Ottawa Charter based themes for health promotion are:

- Building a healthy public policy
- Creating supportive environments
- Developing personal skills
- Strengthening community action
- Reorienting health services towards prevention and health promotion.

These call for a more long term, sustainable approach working in the settings of everyday life. There will be considerable overlap between settings as people move between different sectors as part of daily life.

For each of the interventions provided for the various settings, an example of aims and objectives are included at the end of the chapter for projects that are currently running (Appendix 1). Wherever possible oral health promotion programmes can be closely linked with oral assessment and outreach treatment programmes using mobile dental units.

Oral health promotion in neighbourhoods

There are a range of agencies and projects that are active in many neighbourhoods.

- Sure Start

Including oral health promotion in the multi-agency work of Sure Start working with young children and their families is practised in many areas.

- Traveller Programme

This is an outreach programme working closely with Sure Start, which also has an oral treatment component.

• Healthy Living Centres

Another example of a more generic approach to health, also offers opportunities for including oral health.

• Community Mapping Project

This is an example of a community participation project run by Sustain, an alliance of organisations which promotes better food policy and practice[9].

Oral health promotion in schools

There has been a long tradition of carrying out health education in schools. Oral health is also a topic within the National Curriculum and the 'hidden curriculum' or culture of the school can also influence health behaviour[10]. The school also provides a setting to contact children and parents from pre-school nursery to secondary school. More modern approaches to oral health promotion reach beyond the curriculum and work with schools developing healthy policies and develop the schools links with their local communities. This involves working with schoolteachers, parents and governors, school health nurses and other agencies in the school. Oral health promotion interventions should also be closely linked with the types of oral assessments and screenings of school population. This provides a more co-ordinated approach to the contacts between dental teams and the teaching staff and other health professionals who work in the school setting. Some examples of oral health promotion programmes in school settings include:

• Reception Class intake meetings
• Nursery programme
• Mother and Toddler playgroups
• Educational resources support
• PPA meetings
• Fissure sealant programme
• Smoking cessation programme.

Oral health promotion in the workplace

The enormous range of workplaces provide an opportunity to reach the adult population, many of which do not have regular contact with dental services[11]. Aside from health promotion related to first aid and accident prevention, there are also interventions related to healthy lifestyles and practices being undertaken[12]. Of particular interest to oral health, the workplace often provides a less stressful and more relaxed environment than the clinical setting for oral health promotion interventions.

Workplace oral health promotion programmes can link closely with oral assessment and screening. An example of overlap of the discrete settings in the following examples is the programme for the school workforce as part of the school based fissure sealant programme for children.

- Workplace programme
- Screening and assessment.

Oral health promotion in primary health care and hospitals

The use of the NHS itself as a setting may at first sight seem obvious for any health promotion intervention, but there has been traditionally more concentration on the treatment and curative aspects of health care. But within primary health care there has been a greater focus on health promotion in line with major initiatives such as 'Health for all 2000' from the WHO[13]. Most people contact primary health services at some point in their life. There has been an historical separation of primary dental services from the rest of the primary health care team and the oral health promotion team members offer an opportunity to bridge that gap. As we have reiterated throughout this text, there is a need for all members of the health care team to promote oral health and a key example of an oral health promotion intervention is the education and training in oral care skills for health professionals. The NHS is the UK's largest employer and also provides an opportunity for workplace based interventions.

Some examples of oral health promotion interventions in primary health care and hospitals include:

- Teaching and training oral care skills to health workers
  (See Chapter 7 for a nursing curriculum)
  (Appendix 2 - Case studies for discussion)
- Sugar free prescribing
- Infant feeding policies
- Feeding guidelines for special care groups
- Nutritional policies for hospital catering.

20.8   Summary

There are opportunities for the promotion of oral health using evidence based approaches. Although approaches are sometimes directed by funding associated with specific interventions, a rationale approach to planning and evaluation can be utilised. Historically, the traditional approach to dental health education has often been in isolation of other health education activities. It is now clear that a partnership approach and collaboration with other agencies and teams will yield more effective results.

References

1. Kay E, Locker D. Effectiveness of oral health promotion: a review. London; Health Education Authority, 1997.

2. Sprod A, Anderson A, Treasure ET. Effective Oral Health Promotion Literature Review. Health Promotion Wales Technical Report 20. July 1996. Health Promotion Wales.

3. Batchelor P, Sheiham A. The limitations of a 'high-risk' approach for the prevention of dental caries. *Community Dent Oral Epidemiol* 2002 **30**: 302.

4. Better Health Better Wales. Welsh Assembly Government. 1998.

5. Our Healthier Nation. Dept of Health. 1999.

6. Ewles L, Simnett I. *Promoting Health. A Practical Guide.* 4th Ed. p77. Baillière Tindall, 1999.

7. Ibid. p78

8. Naidoo J, Wills J. *Health Promotion. Foundations for Practice.* 2nd Ed. p261. Baillière Tindall, 2000.

9. Effective oral health promotion through community development. Papers from the Oral Health Promotion Research Group annual conference Oct 2000. Ed. Kwan S, Hamburger R & Weeks J. p24.

10. Cook S A. How does a school based oral health promotion programme affect school teachers and school culture? MSc in Public Health (Health Promoting). Uni West England. Dec 2000.

11. Nuttall N, Steele JG, Nunn J *et al.* A Guide to the UK Adult Dental Health Survey 1998. p35. London: BDA Books, 2001.

12. Naidoo J, Wills J. *Health Promotion. Foundations for Practice.* 2nd Ed. p273. Baillière Tindall, 2000.

13. Ibid. p311.

Appendix I

Gwent Healthcare NHS Trust Community Dental Service

ORAL HEALTH PROMOTION PROGRAMMES 2002

Overall Aims:
- To promote good oral health
- To implement national and local oral health promotion strategies

Overall Objectives:
- Encourage registration with a dentist
- Encourage regular tooth brushing
- Promote the use of fluoride tooth paste
- Reduce the consumption of sugary foods and drinks

Programme Evaluation: Specific outcome measures for individual programmes.

Individual Programme	Target Group
Baby Clinics	0 – 4 children, parents / carers
Sure Start Programmes	0 – 4 children, parents / carers
Teenage Mothers	0 – 4 children, parents / carers
Mother and Toddler Groups	0 – 4 children, parents / carers / group leaders
Healthy Living Centres	Community mothers and support staff
Parent and Playgroup Association	Group leaders
Play Groups	0 – 4 children, parents / carers / group leaders
Nurseries	0 – 4 children, parents / carers / teachers
School Reception Intake	0 – 4 children, parents / carers / teachers
School Screening Assessment	Children, parents / carers
School Resource Support	Children, teachers, support staff
Fissure Sealant Programme	Year 3 pupils, teachers, support staff
Fissure Sealant Programme Phase 2	Year 4, 5, 6 pupils, teachers, support staff
Travellers	Travellers and community mothers
NNEB students	Students, teachers
First year nursing students	Nursing students
Branch programme nursing students	Nursing students
Nursing - Continuing Education	Qualified nurses
Health Visitor Training	Student Health Visitors
Workplaces	Employees
Age Concern	The older person
Crossroads	Respite carers
Nursing, Residential and Care Homes	Carers and managers

Each programme has specific aims and objectives to enable evaluation. For more details, contact: steve.boyle@gwent.wales.nhs.uk

Appendix 2

Case studies

Case studies provide an excellent method of discussing barriers and risk factors for oral health, and identifying the issues for developing a care plan. The following case studies are based on real life examples

Case Study 1	Mrs Kendall
Age	35
Social History	Divorced, lives alone in ground floor flat Studying A level Sociology
Impairment	Registered disabled and receiving benefits Dependent for all activities of daily living and personal needs Wheelchair user including self-propelled electric wheelchair Care provided by 7 carers from different agencies
Communication	Speech unclear. Uses a word board and an electronic voice
Medical history	Cerebral palsy Abnormal swallow Reflux oesophagitis
Medication	Baclofen (to control spasms) Gaviscon (for gastric problems)
Dental status / Dental history	Dentate Received some treatment under GA Bruxism (tendency to grind teeth)
Diet	Soft to facilitate swallowing

Case Study 2	Mr Williams
Age	42
Social History	Lives with elderly parents in family home Attends a Day Centre to develop personal skills Goes into respite care every 6 weeks to give parents a break Registered disabled and receiving benefits Parents are elderly and rather frail
Impairment	Learning difficulty but self-caring Needs prompting with personal hygiene Mobile and can use public transport alone
Communication	No problems. Poor concentration
Medical history	Down syndrome Heart murmur Obesity Epilepsy – well controlled
Medication	Epanutin (anti-convulsant)
Dental status / Dental history	Partially dentate, wears partial upper dentures Prone to gingivitis and periodontal disease Poor oral hygiene Cooperative for dental treatment
Diet	Good appetite, high intake of cakes and biscuits

Case Study 3	Mrs Jones
Age	59
Social History	Lives with husband who has given up work to care for her Sleeps downstairs Waiting for a grant for ground floor shower and toilet Registered disabled and receiving benefits Community Nurse calls daily to assist husband Attends Day Hospital twice a week for physiotherapy
Impairment	Restricted mobility and manual impairment Dependent for personal hygiene Wheelchair user
Communication	Good. Welsh is first language
Medical history	Rheumatoid arthritis affecting all joints Tempero-mandibular joint (TMJ) affected
Medication	Aspirin Steroids
Dental status / Dental history	No teeth in upper arch – Complete upper denture worn Dentate in lower arch – Partial lower denture worn No dental treatment for 3 years Complete upper denture worn at night
Diet	Normal but cut up small

Case Study 4	Susan Davies
Age	3
Social History	Lives with single parent and grandmother Brother and sister aged 5 and 7 years Specialist health visitor calls regularly Family in receipt of benefits
Impairment	Severe learning difficulty due to anoxic brain damage Totally dependent for all aspects of care No mobility
Communication	No speech
Medical history	Anoxic brain damage due to toxaemia in pregnancy Prone to aspiration respiratory infections Epilepsy Vision and hearing affected
Medication	Epanutin (anti-convulsant) Frequent courses of antibiotics for chest infections
Dental status / Dental history	Primary dentition has started to erupt No previous dental attendance
Diet	On food supplements for weight gain

Case Study 5	Mr Marley
Age	57
Social History	British citizen of Afro-caribbean descent Lives in a hostel Regular contact with Community Psychiatric Nurse (CPN) Poor personal hygiene Heavy smoker 'rollies' Occasional cannabis use In receipt of benefits
Impairment	Mental health problems Social exclusion through race and mental illness
Communication	No problems
Medical history	Diagnosis of schizophrenia
Medication	Regular injections of anti-psychotic medication Haloperidol
Dental status / Dental history	Partially dentate Neglected mouth with grossly decayed teeth and periodontal disease. Irregular dental attendance only for pain relief
Diet	Normal but poor quality High fluid a intake, mainly carbonated drinks

Case Study 6	Group home in the community
Residents	5 adults with varying degrees of learning difficulty aged 25 - 52 years Two residents who use wheelchairs are severely physically impaired. The remaining three contribute towards the running of the house under supervision but sometimes need prompting with personal care
Support	Residents supported by a team of care staff who have little training House is managed by a nurse with a qualification in learning disability
Social history	Residents were previously institutionalised Little family contact
Dental status / Dental history	Two of the more able residents wear complete dentures Three residents are dentate and dependent for oral hygiene Irregular dental attendance only for pain relief
Diet	Normal diet Frequent snacks between meals and high intake of carbonated drinks

Identify: **Barriers to oral health**
                             Risk factors for oral health
                             Dietary advice
                             Individual preventive programme
                             Oral health education training needs

Appendix 3

Resources and further reading

Levine R, Stillman-Lowe C. The scientific basis of oral health education. 5th Edition: British Dental Association. 2004.

Nunn J (Editor). Disability and Oral Care. International Association for Disability and Oral Health and FDI. FDI World Dental Press, 2000.

Ireland R (Editor). Advanced Dental Nursing. Blackwell Publishers Ltd. 2004.

Scully C, Cawson R. Medical Problems in Dentistry. 5th Ed. Churchill Livingstone. 2004.

White R (Editor). Trends in Oral Health Care. (BJN Monograph). Mark Allen Publishing Ltd. 2004.

Frude N. Understanding Abnormal Psychology. Blackwell Publishers Ltd. 1998.

Fraser W, Sines D, Kerr M. Hallas. The Care of People with Intellectual Disabilities. 9th Ed. Butterworth-Heinemann 1998.

Atkinson D, Jackson M, Walmsley J. Forgotten Lives. BILD Publications 1997.

Naidoo & Wills Health Promotion. Foundations for Practice. Baillière Tindall 2000

Ewles & Simnett. Promoting Health. A Practical Guide. Baillière Tindall 1999

BSDH Guidelines for Oral Health Care in PDF format on BSDH website:

- Long-stay Patients and Residents
- Dependent, Dysphagic, Critically and Terminally Ill Patients
- Domiciliary Dental Care Services
- Mental Health Problems
- People with a Physical Disability

Also on this website:

- Clinical Guidelines and Integrated Care Pathways for the Oral Health Care of People with a Learning Disability
- Multi-disciplinary Guidelines for the Oral Management of Patients following Oncology Treatment
- Principles on Intervention for People Unable to Comply with Routine Dental Care

Journals

Journal of Disability and Oral Health: Details on BSDH website (see below)
Gerodontology: Details on BSG website (see below)

Web Publications

Essence of Care (2001): www.doh.gov.uk/essenceofcare/index/htm
Fundamentals of Care (2003):
www.wales.gov.uk/subihealth/content/flyer-e.pdf

Websites

British Society for Disability and Oral Health (BSDH):
www.bsdh.org.uk

British Society of Gerodontology (BSG):
http://mysite.wanadoo-members.co.uk/gerodontology

British Fluoridation Society: www.liv.ac.uk/bfs/

International Association for Disability and Oral Health (IADH): www.iadh.org

Disabled People and Carers Information on Employment, Health and Education: www.direct.gov.uk

Disability Rights Commission (DRC): www.drc-gb.org

Disabled Living Foundation (DLF): www.dlf.org.uk

British National Formulary: www.bnf.org

Mun-H-Center: www.mun-h-center.com

The British Council of Disabled People (BCODP): www.bcodp.org.uk

Disability Discrimination Act 1995: www.disability.gov.uk/dda/

Disability Organisations: www.kidsactive.org.uk/dislinks.htm
www.adapttrust.co.uk

Index